# VENOMOUS
# CREATURES
# *of* AUSTRALIA

## Also by S K Sutherland:

*Family Guide to Dangerous Animals and Plants of Australia*

*Australian Animal Toxins. The creatures, their toxins and care of the poisioned patient*

*Take Care. Poisonous Australian Animals*

*Hydroponics for Everyone*

*A Venomous Life*

# VENOMOUS CREATURES
# *of* AUSTRALIA

*A Field Guide with*
*Notes on First Aid*

## Fifth Edition

### Struan K. Sutherland
M.D. (Melb), D.Sc., F.R.A.C.P., F.R.C.P.A.

### John Sutherland
B.Sc. (Melb), LL.B.

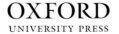

OXFORD
UNIVERSITY PRESS

# OXFORD

253 Normanby Road, South Melbourne, Victoria, Australia

Oxford University Press is a department of the University of Oxford.
It furthers the University's objective of excellence in research, scholarship,
and education by publishing worldwide in

Oxford  New York

Athens  Auckland  Bangkok  Bogotá  Buenos Aires  Calcutta
Cape Town  Chennai  Dar es Salaam  Delhi  Florence  Hong Kong  Istanbul
Karachi  Kuala Lumpur  Madrid  Melbourne  Mexico City  Mumbai  Nairobi
Paris  Port Moresby  São Paulo  Singapore  Taipei  Tokyo  Toronto  Warsaw
with associated companies in  Berlin  Ibadan

OXFORD is a registered trade mark of Oxford University Press
in the UK and certain other countries

First published 1981
Revised edition 1982, Reprinted 1982
Revised editions 1985, Reprinted 1989
Revised edition 1994
Revised edition with John Sutherland 1999

National Library of Australia
Cataloguing-in-Publication data:

Sutherland, Struan, 1936–.
 Venomous creatures of Australia:
 a field guide with notes on first aid

 5th ed.
 Bibliography.
 Includes index.
 ISBN 0 19 550846 7

 1. First aid in illness and injury.
 2. Poisonous animals – Australia. I. Title.

591.650994

Edited and Indexed by David Meagher
Cover and text designed by Steve Randles
Typeset by Derrick Stone
Printed by Craft Print, Singapore

# Contents

## Stinging Fish · 97

## Other Sea Creatures · 119

# Preface

A person aware of the appearance and likely habitat of a venomous creature is less likely to be bitten or stung than the uninformed. Australia is inhabited by some of the most venomous land and sea creatures in the world. This fact, combined with problems of communication, makes a venomous bite or sting potentially all the more dangerous.

All Australians should have some knowledge of the actions of the venoms produced by these animals and the appropriate first aid measures, and this ought to be an essential part of the school curriculum. Not only does this information allow precautions to be taken to avoid bites and stings, but basic first aid may prove to be life saving. Thus the purpose of the book is to bring together excellent illustrations of the most important venomous creatures along with basic facts about each species.

Each creature is illustrated, most in colour. An accompanying map shows the distribution of each animal. Technical terms have been kept to a minimum so that in an emergency a reader may find it as easy as possible to identify the offending creature and understand the type and degree of danger it may present. In some situations the use of scientific terms is necessary — for example, when considering the body scales of snakes. In these situations, we have endeavoured to explain the terms.

Some of the creatures which are known to be dangerous have had little published about them. Rather than omit such animals, they have been included even though the information is sparse.

The publishers asked for a book covering 60 venomous creatures, and the term 'venomous' naturally excludes some very dangerous Australian animals, such as puffer fish (which are poisonous when eaten), sharks and crocodiles. However, there are enough terrors within the covers of this book to keep the reader occupied for the time being! The limitations also mean that some creatures of medical importance, such as mosquitoes and sandflies, have been left out.

None of these venomous creatures have anything to gain by injuring humans. In fact, most go to considerable lengths to avoid confrontation. If you come face to face with any of the creatures illustrated in this book, retreat at once and admire them from a safe distance.

Following requests by health workers to make technical advice more accessible, some such information has been included to assist doctors with patient care (pages 7–10). Subjects briefly dealt with include the administration of antivenoms, tissue damage due to spider bite and the management of fish stings.

   To our delight, this little book continues to spread itself quietly across the country. Incidents have occurred in which the first aid therein has proved life-saving, and some patients have even arrived at hospital clutching a copy! Fortunately this is very rare, as the reader who is careful is almost guaranteed immunity from bites and stings. At least, we hope so.

   Struan K. Sutherland
   John Sutherland
   December 1998

# Acknowledgments

With pleasure we recognise the debt owed to those who have worked on aspects of our venomous wildlife, the venoms, or the management of the envenomed patient.

We appreciate the generosity and unstinted kindness of those listed below. Sadly, some have passed on. The names of such friends are in bold, which is appropriate because they all did bold things in their different ways.

Lyn Abra, Dr Chris Acott, Dr Phil Alderslade, Professor Paul Alewood, Dr Brian Baldo, Chris Banaks, Allen Broad, Professor Kevin Broady, Professor Joseph Burnett, Professor Vic Callanan, Dr Hal Cogger, Neville Coleman, Alan Coulter, Dr Jeanette Covacevich, Dr John Coventry, Professor Bart Currie, Marc Dorse, **Vernon Draffin,** Dr Alan Duncan, Dr Carol Edmonds, **Dr Robert Endean,** Dr Peter Fenner, Professor Malcolm Fisher, Keith Gillett, Graeme Gow, Dr Mike Gray, Professor John Harris, Rodney Harris, Dr Robert Hartwick, Professor Harold Heatwole, Dr Douglas Howarth, Professor Merlin Howden, Dr Bernie Hudson, Professor George Jelinek, Rudie Kuiter, Dr Richard Lewis, Dr Col Limpus, Dr Paul Masci, Professor Dietrich Mebs, Professor Sherman Minton, Peter Mirtschin, Professor John Pearn, Dr Robert Premier, Dr Robert Raven, Dr Jacquie Rifkin, **Dr Ron Southcott,** Dr Bernie Stone, **Charles Tanner,** Dr David Theakston, Professor Tom Torda, Professor Mike Tyler, Dr Ken Walker, Dr Bryan Walpole, Professor David Warrell, John and Robyn Weigel, Dr Julian White, Dr Ian Whyte, Professor John Williamson AM, **Eric Worrell.**

Special mention should be made of help from the Australian Venom Research Unit by Dr Ken Winkel, Dr Gabrielle Hawdon and Vanessa Tresidder.

Dr James Tibballs expertly assisted in the 'fine tuning' of the sections on first aid and medical management.

The encouragement of Professor James Angus and the Honorable Alan Stockdale MP is greatly appreciated.

Finally we thank David Meagher for his meticulous editing of this edition.

# Notes on First Aid
## *for* Bites *and* Stings

The pressure–immobilisation method of first aid described below became the recommended first aid for snake bite in Australia in 1979. In 1980 it was discovered that it also immobilised other types of venom such as that of the Sydney Funnel-web Spider, and it became the standard first aid method for all bites and stings in Australia apart from the exceptions listed on pages 3–5.

## The Pressure–Immobilisation Method of First Aid

The purpose of first aid for most poisonous bites or stings is to stop the venom spreading away from the bitten area and attacking vital parts of the body. If the venom can be kept in one place, the victim may arrive at hospital in good health. Another advantage of effective first aid is that the patient may require far less antivenom when in hospital.

In 1975 the Commonwealth Serum Laboratories (now CSL Ltd) in Melbourne developed a method for measuring snake venom and snake neurotoxins in the blood and tissues of human snake bite victims and experimental animals. This enabled scientists to study how venom moved away from where it had been injected and how it spread through the body. Monkeys were used for much of this work because their limbs are shaped like humans. A monkey would be injected with venom near its ankle, and the rate at which venom moved up the leg and into its blood stream was followed. When the monkey became ill it would be given antivenom and quickly recovered. Using this 'monkey model' various types of first aid were studied and a very simple but safe method was discovered. It was found that if a bandage was wrapped firmly around the leg where the venom was injected, and the leg was kept still, very little venom

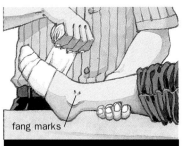

fang marks

**1** Apply a broad pressure bandage over the bite site as soon as possible. (Do not take off jeans as the movement of doing so will assist venom to enter the blood stream. Keep the bitten leg still.)

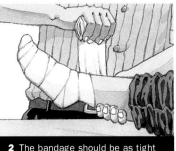

**2** The bandage should be as tight as one you would apply to a sprained ankle.

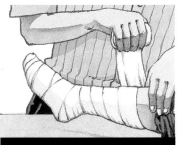

**3** Extend the bandages as high as possible.

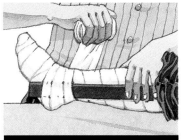

**4** Apply a splint to the leg, immobilising the joints either side of the bite if possible.

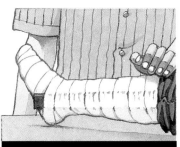

**5** Bind it firmly to elbow with bandages.

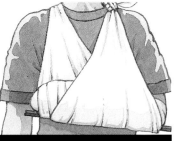

**6** Bites on the hand or forearm. **a** Bind as much of the arm as possible. **b** Use a splint to the elbow. **c** Use a sling.

**Note:** Regardless of the area of the body which has been bitten, **the first aid works better when the victim is kept as still as possible.**

moved up the leg. The venom was trapped under the bandage and stayed put while the bandage was in position. The bandage could be left for hours if necessary and it caused neither pain nor damage to the leg. This method of first aid is potentially life saving.

Snake venom detection kits are now used in most Australian hospitals and allow the doctor to discover quickly the type of snake venom present on clothing, at the bitten area, in blood or in urine (see page 7). It is no longer necessary to kill the snake (and risk further bites) in order to take it to the hospital with the victim.

### Funnel-web Spider bites

Good first aid can be life saving, and everyone living in the Sydney area should be familiar with the pressure–immobilisation method. It has been found that when it is used some of the venom is actually destroyed by the body while it is trapped under the pressure bandage. Thus correct first aid allows the body to destroy the venom (if any has been injected) *and* allows the patient to arrive at a hospital in good health. Fortunately, bites to the body by this spider are rare, so the pressure–immobilisation method of first aid can be used in the majority of cases. First aid measures should be continued in hospital until appropriate drugs and equipment are ready.

# Exceptions to the Pressure–Immobilisation Method of First Aid

### Ant, bee and wasp stings

Remove the insect from the wound. Remove a bee sting and the attached venom sac as quickly as possible. Most stings respond to the application of iced water made by mixing ice and water in a plastic bag. The pressure-immobilisation method should not be used in non-allergic persons as it may prolong the pain of the sting. Medical care should be sought if the reactions are severe. If the victim is known to be highly allergic to these stings, the pressure–immobilisation method should be used to restrict the movement of the venom while the patient is being taken to the doctor. If a severe allergic reaction occurs and breathing and/or the heart stops, give mouth to mouth resuscitation and/or external cardiac compression and summon medical or paramedical aid.

## Red-back Spider bites

The venom of this spider moves very slowly and any attempt to slow it down further increases pain so no restrictive bandages should be used. No first aid is required. Seek medical aid at once. Take along the spider in a jar for positive identification. Iced water (made by mixing ice and water in a plastic bag) may reduce the pain if it is applied to the bitten area — but do not freeze the skin.

## Australian Paralysis Tick bites

It is essential that the tick (or ticks) be removed as quickly and as gently as possible. Those that have been on the body for only a few hours are easily wiped off. Ticks that are well buried may have to be lifted out using a pair of sharp-pointed scissors. The aim is to extract the whole tick in one piece, including its mouth parts. Avoid squeezing the tick, as more poison may be introduced into the victim. Do not apply kerosene, ether, or other chemicals that would irritate the tick, as this will make it insert more toxin. Once the tick has been removed the patient will start improving. The pressure–immobilisation method can be used *after* the tick has been extracted. Only very ill patients need antitoxin.

## Box Jellyfish stings

Pour domestic vinegar or dilute acetic acid (never spirits or other types of alcohol) over the adhering tentacles to inactivate them before trying to remove them. After five minutes they can be wiped off with a dry towel. Tentacles should never be wiped with clothing or sand before they have been inactivated by vinegar, as this will only trigger off more stinging capsules. Take the victim to a doctor or hospital. If the victim's breathing and/or heartbeat is failing, give mouth to mouth resuscitation and/or external cardiac massage and summon medical or paramedical aid. Hospitals in the sub-tropical regions of Australia stock Box Jellyfish antivenom. This antivenom has proved very satisfactory in a number of critically ill victims, and also reduces the disfiguring skin changes which may occur.   ·

## Other jellyfish stings

Some jellyfish stings, such as those due to the Irukandji and the Jimble, should be treated with vinegar or dilute acetic acid, as for Box Jellyfish stings. If the reaction is severe, take the victim to a doctor or hospital. In most cases there is plenty of time to reach medical aid.

Sometimes powerful pain killers may be required. Current opinion is that vinegar should not be used for most other jellyfish stings such as those due to Blue-bottles or Sea Blubbers. These should be treated with iced water or wrapped ice cubes.

### Stinging fish, especially stonefishes

The only stinging fishes for which an antivenom is available are the stonefishes. First aid for a fish sting is as follows:

**1** Relieve the pain. This is usually best and most effectively produced by drug therapy by a medical practitioner. Local anaesthetic and/or opiates may be required in severe cases.

**2** If medical aid is not available immediately, bathe the wound in water which is warm enough to be effective but not scald the skin. Many fish venoms are thought to be inactivated by warm to hot water. The heat also increases the blood flow in the injured area, thus dispersing the venom throughout the blood stream. Most of the effects of the venom occur around the sting, so if the concentration of venom is decreased the local effects are less severe. Pressure–immobilisation techniques are not recommended for use over the stung area, because delaying the movement of venom into the blood stream will only enhance the pain of the sting.

## The Old Type of First Aid

The old methods of first aid were dangerous, often very painful, and could only be used for a very short time.

For many years people were taught to cut into the area that had been bitten in order to get rid of the venom. This was pretty severe treatment, as only small amounts of venom could be removed that way and snakes often inject little or no venom, even though fang marks may be clearly visible.

The next change to the first aid involved the use of arterial tourniquets (which nowadays should *never* be used to treat bites). If someone was bitten by a dangerous snake or spider, say on the foot, then the blood supply to the leg was stopped as soon as possible. The problems associated with arterial tourniquets are threefold:

• They can only be used for a short time because the tissues of the leg start dying after about 20 minutes due to lack of oxygen.

• They can cause severe damage to nerves and arteries, or even to the whole leg.

• They are terribly painful; few people can stand them for long.

# Notes *for* Doctors *and* Paramedical Staff

## Hospital Staff

(See also books listed on page 127.)
Please note that first aid measures are usually removed soon after the patient is admitted. Do not leave them on for hours! The doctor will decide when to remove the bandages. If venom has been injected it will move into the bloodstream very quickly when the bandages are removed, so the doctor should leave them in position until the appropriate antivenom and drugs are assembled for use when the dressings and splints are removed.

## Notes on Antivenoms

Detailed information on the use of antivenoms is packaged with the individual antivenoms. If doctors require appropriate consultants, they can be contacted via the Poisons Information Centres (**131126** Australia wide). Doctors may also contact the medical staff of the Australian Venom Research Unit directly on **(03) 9483-8204** or CSL Ltd on **(03) 9389-1911**.

Australia is the only country in the world that has snake venom detection kits. A swab from the bite site, blood, or urine allows the doctor to select the type of snake antivenom which *may* have to be used. Only one in ten cases of snake bite need antivenom because often the snake injects very little venom.

Antivenoms therefore should not be given unless there is evidence of significant poisoning. For example, in snake bites, signs of systemic poisoning such as nausea, vomiting, ptosis, etc., or positive laboratory findings such as a coagulation defect. Fang marks alone are not an indication for antivenom. Likewise, if the only problem after a Red-back Spider bite is moderate local pain, then antivenom is not indicated at that stage.

Australian antivenoms are established as the safest in the world. Provided they are administered with appropriate premedication, there is no reason for them to be withheld even if the patient has a past history of reaction to equine proteins. These patients, such as snake handlers who have suffered reactions in the past, have had minimal or no problems with repeat antivenom therapy after appropriate premedication.

### Administration of antivenoms

Most antivenoms are given by the intravenous route (see CSL's Product Leaflets). Skin testing with antivenom for allergy to antivenom is unreliable and a waste of time. It may also delay urgent therapy.

It is wise to give premedication before most antivenoms. Patients should receive 0.25 mg of adrenaline by the subcutaneous route (0.005–0.01 mg/kg for a child). The adrenaline premedication should *never* be given intravenously, especially in a normotensive patient. An antihistamine may also be given parenterally, bearing in mind it may have sedatory effects and may also cause hypotension. If the patient has a known history of reacting to antivenoms, then steroids should also be administered. Antivenoms which are to be given intravenously should be diluted 1 in 10. Note that the antivenom requirements of patients will vary considerably. Some patients with minimal envenoming will require no antivenom, whereas others may require multiple doses of antivenom.

Both the incidence and severity of delayed serum sickness may be markedly reduced by the administration of prednisolone 50 mg (adult dose) for five days after the administration of antivenoms.

# Venom Allergy and Anaphylaxis

Patients who have developed severe allergies to either Honey Bee or wasp venom should be referred to an allergist. They may greatly benefit from a series of small injections of purified venom which will convert them from being dangerously allergic to 'immune'. Persons allergic to ant venom should also be referred to an allergist so that they may, if indicated, receive ant venom therapy when it becomes available.

The cornerstone of anaphylaxis management is adrenaline. It should be injected promptly and before any other drug. Patients with known venom allergies should be supplied with adrenaline and they and their family instructed as to the dose to give and how to inject it subcutaneously or intramuscularly. If bronchospasm occurs after envenomation, an aerosol bronchodilator like salbutamol may be helpful, but neither this nor antihistamines should take the place of adrenaline. It should be noted that some snake handlers who have suffered bites in the past have developed dangerous allergies to the snake venoms involved. The injection of a small amount of snake venom may produce a life-threatening reaction. If such individuals are envenomated they require dual treatment: management of anaphylaxis closely, followed by antivenom therapy

## Necrotising Arachnidism

Cyanotic lesions which sometimes occur after spider bites may ulcerate. There is no specific treatment currently available to treat these lesions, which may be extremely painful. Pain relief and bed rest with elevation of the affected area should be instituted. Overseas experience suggests that neither heparin nor high doses of steroids produce any significant improvement. The use of hyperbaric oxygen therapy might be considered. Another therapy to consider is the use of local or general vasodilators. Most patients are put on antibiotics without apparent effect on the lesions.

Slowly spreading ulcers are sometimes found to be due to *Mycobacterium ulcerans*, which responds to appropriate therapy.

## Fish and Stingray Stings

### Pain relief

Pain relief is obtained quickly by bathing the injured region in warm, but not scalding, water. If necessary, boat-engine cooling water can be used. Often the pain returns quite dramatically when the heat therapy is stopped.

Local anaesthetic agents are sometimes indicated and, in severe cases, a regional nerve block by means of bupivacaine or lignocaine may be necessary.

Systemic opiate therapy may be required.

Antivenom should be administered with appropriate precautions in significant stonefish stings.

## Care of the injured area

Take positive action and remove foreign bodies or dead tissues. Local tissue necrosis is usual with envenomation by stingray spines. Ensure good drainage. X-ray examination may be necessary.

Wash very well with fresh water, as sea water may encourage bacterial growth. The wound is potentially infected, so remember that marine bacteria represent a wide range of organisms, many of which are not characterised fully. Most are resistant to common antibiotic agents, and also require special salinated media for culture. Expert opinion is that doxycycline is the drug of first choice.

## General effects

- Maintain vital functions (ABC — airway, breathing and circulation).
- Shock — note pain relief as above.
- Effects of venom — antivenom if indicated.

## Note

With the exception of bites by blue-ringed octopuses, cone shell stings and sea-snake bites, the pressure–immobilisation technique should not be used to attempt to hold marine toxins at the site of the bite or sting. To do so may increase pain and local tissue damage.

## Additional note

Tetanus prophylaxis should be updated as required. (Death from tetanus has occurred after stingray injuries.)

It may be necessary to rest the injured region for days for satisfactory healing to occur.

# Snakes

# Introduction

There are over 100 species of snakes in Australia, of which some 25 species may be considered dangerous to man. This is a very high proportion of venomous snakes compared with other countries. Globally there are some 3000 different species of snakes and the vast majority of these are harmless to man. All the dangerous snakes in Australia belong to the elapid family and are front fanged. A number of these are world leaders in total poison output. They produce highly poisonous venom, often in very large quantities. The potentially most venomous snake in the world is the Small-scaled or Fierce Snake (No. 14), and the next eight place-getters are also Australian.

Snakes are cold-blooded, and their degree of activity is usually related to the surrounding temperature. Most snakes hibernate in the cooler months but the hibernation is not complete. An Australian snake disturbed in winter is perfectly capable of becoming extremely active and inflicting a bite.

## Senses

All snakes are completely deaf, but they can detect the movement of creatures by vibrations on the ground which are transmitted through the snake's body.

The vision of snakes is not very good, and often a snake will not notice an object until it moves. They have no eyelids, but each eye is covered by a scale which is normally transparent. However, when the skin is being shed this eye scale becomes opaque, and for a day or so the snake will have clouded vision. The absence of an eyelid accounts for the snake's fixed beady stare which people often find so horrifying.

All snakes have an excellent sense of smell. They use their forked tongues to pick up tiny particles from the ground and transfer them to two pits called Jacobson's organs, which are sensitive smelling organs situated in the roof of their mouth. This is why a snake flicks its tongue to the ground and in and out of the mouth as it moves along. The snake can also smell through its nostrils, but not very efficiently.

## Shedding of the skin (sloughing)

Snakes slough their outer skins quite regularly. This happens more frequently in the younger, faster-growing snakes, and is more common in warm weather. In the normal course of sloughing, first the scale covering the eye becomes cloudy, and after several days this clears and then the snake will look for some object to rub against to assist in extricating itself from the old skin. The skin over the snout and lips is first pushed back and turned over the head. The old skin is then turned inside out like the removal of a stocking. A snake which has recently shed its skin is usually at its most colourful. Incidentally, the skin of a snake is not slimy, as is often believed, but is quite dry.

## Movement

Snakes are slow-moving creatures, with a maximum speed on level ground of about 7 km per hour. They need to grip the surface in order to move forward, so on smooth surfaces such as a sheet of glass they are unable to progress. Although their speed is limited on the ground, if they are held ineffectively by the body they are capable of extremely rapid movement around the point at which they are being held.

The spine of a snake contains from 180 to 400 vertebrae. There is no chest bone, and a pair of ribs is attached to each vertebra by a ball and socket joint. It is the combination of many vertebrae and these ribs which give the snake its flexibility and rapid speed over short distances. When a snake moves, each part of the body follows the same winding course. All snakes can swim, and those that feed on frogs and eels are very often found swimming in rivers and dams.

## Reproduction

Of the highly dangerous snakes, only the Taipan (No. 13), Small-scaled Snake (No. 14), Mulga Snake (No. 9) and brown snakes (Nos 3-6) lay eggs. All others bear live young, although some young may be born in a thin delicate sac from which they soon escape.

Sometimes when a female snake is killed, these unborn snakes can be seen escaping from the damaged mother's body, and this has led to the mistaken belief that the mother snake, if alarmed, will swallow her young alive to protect them. However, most snakes love eating other snakes, even their young, and once a snake is swallowed it becomes a meal!

## Identification of snakes

Except for the classically coloured Mainland Tiger Snake (No. 1) and the Red-bellied Black Snake (No. 8), colour is a poor means of positively identifying most of the dangerous Australian snakes. In some species, such as the Death Adder (No. 12), the shape of the body is so characteristic that identification is straightforward, but for the majority of the dangerous snakes an examination of the head shields and

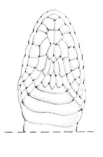
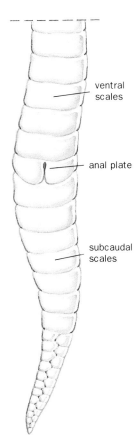

ventral scales

anal plate

subcaudal scales

**Figure 1** The under or ventral surface of a dangerous snake showing the position of the various scales.

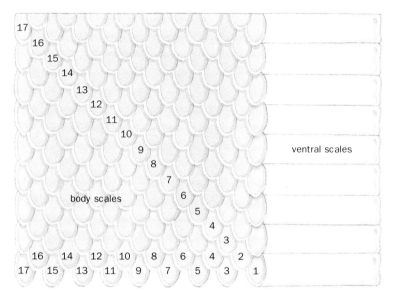

**Figure 2** How body scales are counted. In this example, a piece of skin has been removed from the mid-body of the Common Brown Snake and spread out flat. To remove the skin, the edges of scale 17 were cut where they joined the ventral scales.

the counting of body scales is the only positive way in which definite identification can be made. The important scales are the body scales (which are counted diagonally) and the ventral and subcaudal scales (see Figures 1 and 2). An examination of the anal plate to determine whether it is divided or not is often of key importance. Sometimes scale counting may prove quite difficult because of subtle variations not apparent to the amateur. Indeed, quite skilled snake experts have sometimes made important errors in snake identification.

**Note:** Snake venom detection kits which are held by most hospitals have proved very valuable in selecting the type of antivenom which may have to be used.

## Venom apparatus

The fangs of the Australian venomous snakes are hollow so that the venom (which is produced in two large glands in the sides of the head, behind the eyes) may pass forward through a duct into a canal in the fang and thus be injected from near the tip of the fang in the most efficient way (see Figure 3). When a snake bites, it can control the amount of venom it injects by the degree that the muscles contract around the venom glands. Some snakes hold on and chew when they bite, and this chewing action usually results in large amounts of venom being injected. The fangs of the dangerous Australian snakes are not as mobile as some of the overseas ones, but they do rotate forward to some extent. The most effective envenomation apparatus is found in the Death Adder (No. 12), whose fangs move quite significantly. The fangs of snakes are replaced from time to time, and quite often only one functioning fang may be present because the replacement fang on the other side has not yet moved into position. It is thus possible for humans to be effectively poisoned when only one fang mark can be seen. It is very important to know that, by and large, the fangs of the dangerous Australian snakes are sharply pointed and quite thin. Thus, effective snake poisoning can often occur even though it may be very difficult to see any fang marks.

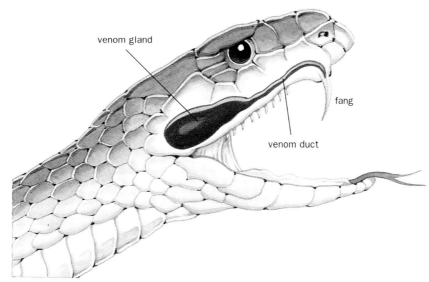

**Figure 3** Head of a snake dissected to show the venom gland and the duct which enters the fang.

## Snake venom

The prime purpose of venom is to enable the snake to paralyse its prey rapidly so it can be swallowed. The major Australian snake venoms contain large amounts of very strong neurotoxins which, when injected into an animal, move around the body and home in on the ends of nerves just where they make contact with the muscles. As a result, the muscles can no longer be stimulated by the nerves, so the animal can neither move nor breathe and the snake's dinner is served! These neurotoxins are proteins, and their structure is well known in the case of certain snake venoms. Some venoms, such as those of tiger snakes (Nos 1 and 2), have three quite separate neurotoxins, each capable of causing paralysis. Some neurotoxins can also directly damage the muscles of the body.

Snake venoms are a complicated mixture of poisons. Apart from neurotoxins there may be a number of other dangerous proteins. One component may disrupt the normal clotting mechanism of blood, so that the wounds continue to bleed instead of stopping after a few minutes as they would normally do. Some proteins damage the red cells in the blood, while others are spreading factors which assist the movement of venom away from the bitten area.

No one knows why Australian snakes produce so much venom. For example, the average amount of venom produced when the snake expert milks a Taipan (No. 13) is enough to kill 12 000 guinea pigs! It is possible that, because the fangs of the Australian snakes are relatively small and not ideal for holding on to large struggling animals, a means of producing rapid paralysis has been developed.

## Comparisons between the 'killing power' of different snake venoms: the $LD_{50}$

Mice are commonly used to compare the strength of various venoms. The term Lethal Dose 50 per cent of $LD_{50}$ is frequently used and indicates the dose of venom which would kill 50 per cent of a group of mice. Provided enough mice are used and the quantities of venom injected is suitably selected, it is possible to obtain an accurate, reproducible $LD_{50}$ for a venom. This allows it to be compared with other venoms. For example, in mice weighing 18 to 21 grams, the subcutaneous* $LD_{50}$ of Mainland Tiger Snake venom is 2.35 µg[†] but the $LD_{50}$ of the American Diamondback Rattlesnake (*Crotalus adamanteus*) is 228 µg. Thus the $LD_{50}$ test indicates that the venom of the tiger snake is about 100 times more toxic in mice than the most important snake of the United States of America.

Instead of expressing an $LD_{50}$ as the dose for a single mouse it is now more usual to define the dose in milligrams per kilogram body weight of mice, the $LD_{50}$ of 2.35 (g per mouse will become 0.118 mg/kg of mice. Thus if we consider that 50 mice of 18 to 21 gram body weight make a kilogram of mice, the $LD_{50}$ of 2.35 µg per mouse will become 0.118 mg/kg of mice. The preferred mg/kg $LD_{50}$ definition is used throughout this book.

## Feeding habits

Snakes usually swallow a victim's head first, as this gives an easier passage by minimising obstructions. When swallowed this way the limbs or feathers flatten against the body of the victim, streamlining it. Unlike lizards, the lower jaw of the snake can dislocate while the prey is being swallowed, permitting the passage of quite bulky objects. After swallowing its prey, the snake relocates its jaw by a number of opening and closing motions. The

---

* 'subcutaneous' means injected under the skin
† µg = microgram = one millionth of a gram

brain of the snake is enclosed completely by bone, giving it some protection if an animal struggles while being swallowed.

Behind the poison fangs are a number of teeth which curve backwards and prevent the prey moving in any direction except towards the snake's stomach. The digestive juices in a snake's stomach only work properly when the temperature of the snake itself is high enough. If the temperature of the environment (and hence that of the snake) falls to a low level, digestion stops and the swallowed prey may ferment, thus killing the snake. This is a common reason why snakes die in captivity when there is poor temperature control of their cages. The parts of the prey like the hair, claws, feathers and tough skin which are not entirely digested are either excreted or disgorged.

## Preventing snake bite

Snakes have nothing to gain by biting humans, and as a general rule will go to considerable lengths to avoid confronting them. Most bites occur when a human either treads upon or touches a retreating or sleeping snake, which then responds to defend itself. Many snake bites can be avoided if people leave snakes alone, particularly sleeping snakes which may be unaware of a human's presence. Bites often occur when people put their hands in hollow logs or thick grass without looking first. It is important to wear stout shoes and adequate clothing in country where they may be snakes, and people should never wear sandals or thongs in thick grass, along river banks, or in other areas that may be frequented by snakes. It is a wise precaution to keep grass well cut around places like playgrounds and vacant allotments in order to minimise the chance of snakes coming into the area.

On warm summer nights a number of dangerous snakes are active. It is sensible always to use a torch around camps and farm buildings. When snakes approach houses, barns, or chicken sheds they are usually in search of mice and rats, so it is very important to keep the rat and mouse population down.

# 1  Mainland Tiger Snake

## *Notechis scutatus*

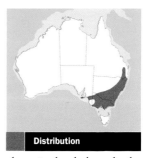

**Distribution**

This snake is a common cause of serious snake bite in Australia. Its natural distribution is near areas of dense population, and people often come across them because of their particular habits. On warm summer evenings, Mainland Tiger Snakes roam around farms and the back lawns of outer suburban houses. They hunt frogs along river banks and around dams, and may enter sheds, kitchens, and even bedrooms after mice. Some people have stood on a snake on a lawn in the dark, and others have been bitten inside buildings. To avoid bites it is very important to take special care and use a torch on warm summer evenings.

The Mainland Tiger Snake is solidly built with a broad head which is hardly distinct from its body, unlike the Taipan (No. 13) which has a distinct and delicate neck. Its average length is 1 metre. The 'classic' tiger snake may be pale brown or almost black, and crossed with about 45

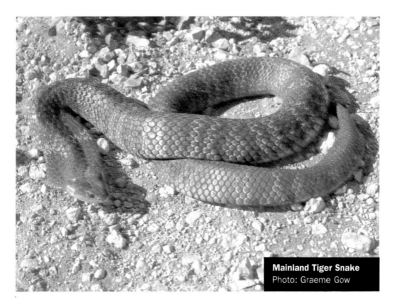

**Mainland Tiger Snake**
Photo: Graeme Gow

yellowish bands. The colour may vary considerably from one district to another, and sometimes the snake has no bands. Some deaths have occurred when someone has been bitten by an unbanded tiger snake and mistaken it for a Common Brown Snake — and hence got the wrong antivenom.

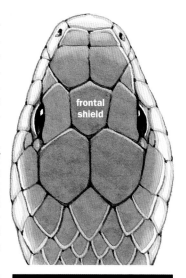

The Mainland Tiger Snake has a wide shield, which is the central one of three between the eyes, and if its colour is unusual this frontal shield may help identify it. The Mainland Tiger snake has 19 rows of mid-body scales; ventrals may be 140 to 190, and subcaudals are 35 to 65 and single, as is the anal plate.

The young are born free and usually number about 30 in a litter.

Mainland Tiger Snakes are generally not aggressive unless provoked. How-

**Head of a Mainland Tiger Snake from above. The characteristic frontal shield is marked.**

ever, if cornered, struck or trodden upon, a ferocious attack may occur. Before striking, the snake flattens its neck. It tends to strike low to the ground, usually not much higher than 30 cm. The average length of its fangs is 3.5 mm and the maximum length recorded is 5.5 mm.

The venom of the Mainland Tiger Snake is the fourth most poisonous in the world, and is present in large quantities. When Mainland Tiger Snakes are milked for their venom, the average yield is 35 mg. The record yield is 180 mg, recorded in 1934; this would kill more than 40 000 adult mice. The $LD_{50}$ of the venom is 0.118 mg/kg in 18 to 21 g mice. The venom contains many separate toxins. It has three types of toxins (neurotoxins) which attack nerve endings, and one of them also damages the muscles. Death is usually due to these neurotoxins. The victim becomes paralysed and cannot breathe, or suffers widespread muscle damage leading to kidney failure and death. Apart from neurotoxins, another toxin prevents blood from clotting properly, so that the victim can bleed to death, but this is very rare.

 Tiger snake antivenom is available to treat bites by this snake.

 First Aid, see pages 1–2

# 2 Black Tiger Snakes

## *Notechis ater*

The Black or Island Tiger Snakes are quite distinct from the Mainland Tiger Snake and show a considerable variation in size, habits and venom. With the exception of the Black Tiger Snakes found in the south-western part of Western Australian and a small area of South Australia (Krefft's Tiger Snake), the species lives only on the islands off the south coast of Australia and in Tasmania. Variations between the different Island Tiger Snakes have evolved since the islands became separated from the mainland.

Black Tiger Snakes have a scattered distribution. In the south-western part of Australia the Western Tiger Snake or Norne (*Notechis ater occidentalis*) is found south of the Moore River but not east of the Stirling Ranges. In the Flinders Ranges there is a small subspecies of Black Tiger Snake called Krefft's Tiger Snake (*Notechis ater ater*). Black Tiger Snakes are also found on the Yorke and Eyre Peninsulas and on Kangaroo Island (the Peninsula Tiger Snake, *Notechis ater niger*) and many of the neighbouring islands. In Bass Strait there are two distinct subspecies. On King Island and most of the Bass Strait islands, *Notechis ater humphreysi* is found, while Chappell and Badger Islands have a larger subspecies, *Notechis ater serventyi*.

Black Tiger Snakes are usually found on the coast or in marshlands. The only form which prefers arid areas is Krefft's Tiger Snake. Usually they are only active in the day. The island snakes eat mostly mutton-birds and frequently live in their burrows.

It is not known how many people have died following bites from these snakes. Certainly a number of mutton-birders have received bites while pulling mutton-birds out of burrows the birds were sharing with a snake. Because of the distance from doctors or hospitals, great care should be taken by visitors to these islands.

These snakes are normally black except for the bellies, which are usually grey. In the Western Australian specimens narrow yellow bands one scale wide are sometimes seen in the adults. In all other subspecies, banding is seen only rarely in immature snakes. The maximum length varies considerably with the subspecies. The longest Black Tiger Snake is the Chappell Island Tiger Snake, which may reach 2.4 metres.

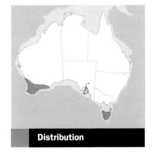

**Distribution**

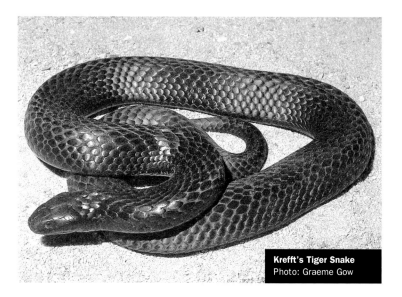

**Krefft's Tiger Snake**
Photo: Graeme Gow

The smallest is Krefft's Tiger Snake, which rarely exceeds 0.9 of a metre. Black Tiger Snakes have 17 or 19 rows of mid-body scales with 155 to 190 ventrals. Subcaudals number 40 to 60 and are all divided, as is the anal plate.

The young of the Black Tiger Snake are born alive with a litter size of 20 to 30 snakes. One specimen from Tasmania was found to contain 109 young.

The Chappell Island Tiger Snake is the most prolific venom producer of all the tiger snakes. The average yield on milking is 74 mg and the maximum yield recorded is 388 mg. The venom of the Chappell Island Tiger Snake is less poisonous than the Mainland Tiger Snake (0.338 mg/kg vs 0.118 mg/kg). However, the venom from the snakes on islands off South Australia is often more poisonous than the Mainland Tiger Snake, and their average yield is 34 mg, which is similar to the Mainland Tiger Snakes.

Black Tiger Snake venom is basically similar to Mainland Tiger Snake venom, causing paralysis and damage to the blood clotting mechanism. Because of the large potential venom output of the Chappell Island Tiger Snake, a person who is bitten by this snake and needs treatment should be given twice the starting dose of tiger snake antivenom that would be given for a Mainland Tiger Snake bite.

 Tiger snake antivenom is available to treat bites by this snake.

 First Aid, see pages 1–2

# 3 Common *or* Eastern Brown Snake

## *Pseudonaja textili*

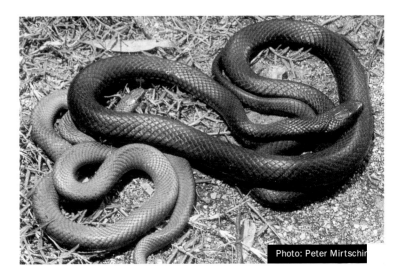

Photo: Peter Mirtschir

The Common Brown Snake is the most frequent cause of death from snake bite in Australia. It is found in a wide area of eastern Australia, from Cape York Peninsula to the Gulf of St Vincent. Three isolated populations occur in the Northern Territory, extending to the north-east corner of Western Australia. It is not found in Tasmania nor on any of the islands off the coast. It has been reported in New Guinea, but it is believed that it was introduced there by man.

The Common Brown Snake feeds on rats, mice, lizards, other snakes and small birds, and is often found around barns and farm houses. It is active by day. Where this snake is common, it is important to keep barns and outbuildings free from rats and mice. Unlike tiger snakes, it prefers dry country to swampy areas.

Common Brown Snakes have a slender streamlined body, and the head is not distinct. The adult is usually uniform in colour, being light brown, orange or black. The young snake may have as many as 50 dark grey or black bands, as well as a broad dark band on the back of its neck. However, strongly banded and unbanded specimens have been found in the same clutch. By the time the snake is 3 years old the bands have disappeared. The average minimum length is less than 1.5 metres and the maximum

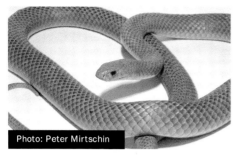

Photo: Peter Mirtschin

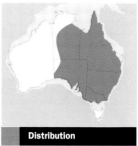

Distribution

recorded is 2.4 metres. The scales are smooth and there are 17 mid-body rows. There are 185 to 235 to ventral scales and the paired subcaudals number 45 to 75. The anal plate is divided. This snake lays from 10 to 35 eggs.

The Common Brown Snake differs from other dangerous Australian snakes in a number of ways. It is active only during the day except when the weather has been extremely hot. When it bites a small animal it winds itself around the creature and holds on until the animal has become paralysed. Prior to attacking, it curves itself into an S shape, raising its head high off the ground. Because of this, people are often bitten above the knee. It only slightly flattens its neck when angry and, when it strikes, it strikes with its mouth wide open, probably because it possesses very short fangs. It can be extremely fast and very ferocious if cornered. Its speed often results in a series of bites being inflicted.

The Common Brown Snake is not a copious venom producer. The average yield is 7 mg and the maximum yield recorded is some 67 mg. The larger brown snakes in Queensland have a higher average yield than the overall eastern Australian average. The venom is very toxic; in fact, it is the second most toxic land snake venom in the world. The subcutaneous $LD_{50}$ for 18 to 21 g mice is 0.053 mg/kg. The venom is extremely neurotoxic and can also rapidly upset the blood clotting mechanism. It does not seem to attack the muscles of the body.

People bitten by a Common Brown Snake may become ill quite rapidly. A severe headache often develops within 15 minutes, and frequently the blood does clot by 30 minutes.

Paralysis develops very slowly and the majority of patients receive antivenom before much paralysis has occurred. The clotting defects may require a large amount of antivenom and other treatment for complete cure. Some people have died because of the clotting defect rather than the paralysis.

 **Common Brown Snake antivenom is available to treat bites by this snake.**

 **First Aid, see pages 1–2**

# Western Brown Snake *or* Gwardar

## *Pseudonaja nuchalis*

The wide distribution of the Western Brown Snake, which overlaps into the territory of the Common Brown Snake, ensures that brown snakes in one form or another are found in most areas of the continent. This snake is distributed throughout Australia but is not found in Tasmania, nor in a broad strip along the eastern coast of Australia extending from the far north into South Australia.

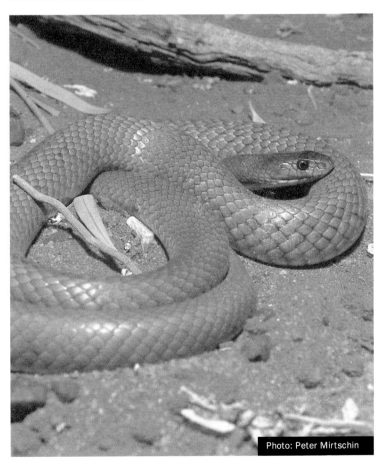

Photo: Peter Mirtschin

The Western Brown Snake is usually active only during the day and its habits and diet are similar to the Common or Eastern Brown Snake (No. 3). However, it is not considered to be as aggressive as that snake.

Like the other members of the *Pseudonaja* genus, this snake has a small head that is indistinct from its body, which is quite slender. It is usually coloured an olive brown or a darkish brown. Sometimes the

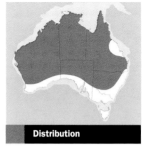

**Distribution**

head is black, and some specimens have a number of broad bands. The belly is usually a light yellowish-cream with light pink or grey spots. The mature snake may grow to a length of 1.5 metres. There are 17 rows of mid-body scales and the ventrals number 184 to 225. The anal plate is divided, as are the 53 to 65 subcaudals.

Females lay an average of 20 eggs a season.

Upon milking, the Western Brown Snake yields an average of some 3 mg of venom which is powerfully neurotoxic and may cause severe disorders of blood clotting. However, its venom is considerably less poisonous in mice than is the Eastern Brown Snake venom, having a subcutaneous $LD_{50}$ in 18 to 21 g mice of 0.47 mg/kg.

Even small snakes can produce quite severe illness. For example, a snake collector was bitten by a specimen which was less than 30 cm long. He ignored the bite because he considered a snake of that size to be harmless. However, within 30 minutes he had developed a severe headache and in an hour was short of breath. He suddenly collapsed and was unconscious for 15 minutes. Upon recovering consciousness, he suffered from blurred vision and marked weakness. For the next 2 days he remained moderately ill and the bite was itchy and tender.

**Common Brown Snake antivenom is available to treat bites by this snake.**

**First Aid, see pages 1–2**

# 5 Dugite

*Pseudonaja affinis*

This snake is frequently a cause of serious snake bite, but it seems to be found only in the southern coastal strip of Western Australia. The Dugite lives in areas of extensive human habitation and often enters houses in search of mice and lizards. It is considered more nervous and aggressive than the Western Brown Snake.

This snake has the small head and typically slender body of the brown snake family. Its back is usually an olive green but may be a dark olive brown. Many specimens are spotted with black flecks and have a dark belly instead of the olive or yellow belly seen in other brown snakes. The belly is often spotted with light pink or grey spots. The Dugite has more body scales than the Common Brown Snake. There are 19 rows of mid-body scales and 190 to 230 ventral scales, and both the anal plate and the 50 to 70 subcaudals scales are divided.

The average yield on milking the Dugite is some 6 mg and the highest venom yield recorded is 17 mg. The subcutaneous $LD_{50}$ dose in 18 to 21 g mice is 0.66 mg/kg. The venom is neurotoxic and may affect the victim's blood clotting.

Persons bitten by this snake who are effectively envenomed and do not receive adequate first aid may develop signs of poisoning within 15 minutes of being bitten. The clotting disturbances can be so severe that the victim has a high risk of suffering a massive haemorrhage.

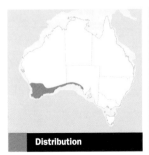

Distribution

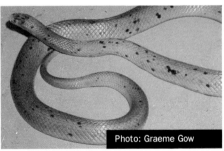

Photo: Graeme Gow

 Common Brown Snake antivenom is the antivenom of choice.

 First Aid, see pages 1–2

# 6  Speckled Brown Snake

## *Pseudonaja guttata*

This snake is limited to an area in central Queensland and part of the Northern Territory. It is active during the day and shelters down deep earth cracks. It is commonly encountered near lakes and dams, where it feeds mainly on frogs.

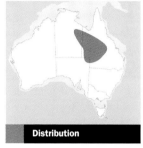

**Distribution**

The Speckled Brown Snake has the typical build of a brown snake. Its back is normally a light brown or cream with some scales showing black margins. However, banded forms are also known. The belly is light yellow with orange spots. The maximum recorded length is 1.25 metres. The body scales are in 21 rows, the ventrals number 204, and the 60 subcaudals are divided. The anal plate is also divided.

Very little is known about this snake. It is highly strung, like all brown snakes, but it is not very aggressive. Studies have shown that the subcutaneous $LD_{50}$ of this venom in 18 to 21 g mice is 0.36 mg/kg. It should be considered a highly dangerous snake.

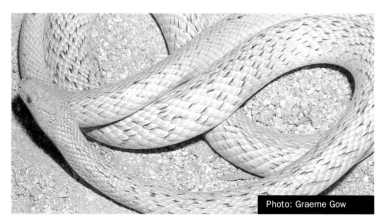

Photo: Graeme Gow

Common Brown Snake antivenom neutralises the venom of this snake.

First Aid, see pages 1–2

# 7  Copperhead

*Austrelaps superbus*

This snake is highly venomous but fortunately, because of its unaggressive nature, rarely bites humans. The Copperhead is found only in south-eastern Australia and Tasmania. Its distribution includes the highlands of New South Wales and through Victoria as far as the Mount Lofty Ranges and Kangaroo Island. It is also found on some of the Bass Strait islands. Some experts believe there are two subspecies of the Copperhead.

The Copperhead prefers a cool climate and on very cold days may be out hunting. On hot days it does most of its hunting at night. It can even be found above the snow line on Mt. Kosciusko. Copperheads often congregate around swamps, rivers and creeks. They feed upon frogs, reptiles and small mammals. They will eat other snakes and often eat their own young. They have a short hibernation which is usually spent underground.

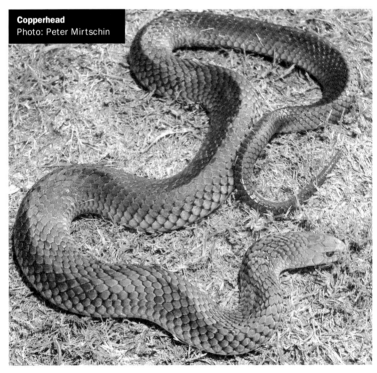

Copperhead
Photo: Peter Mirtschin

The Copperhead is more solidly built than the Mainland Tiger Snake (No. 1). Its small head is slightly distinct from the neck and most Copperheads, especially in New South Wales, have a characteristically striped upper lip. The stripes are usually alternating white and brown. The colour of the body is very variable. It may be dark brown or black or an attractive rich, light copper. Often there is a dark stripe on the back and some-

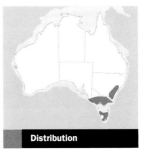

**Distribution**

times a dark collar on the back of the neck, which usually has a yellow border. This is more common in young snakes. The two outer rows of large scales on the flanks may be pink or red, creating a red stripe down the side; Copperheads which have red stripes may be mistaken for Red-bellied Black Snakes. The belly may be bright yellow, cream or light grey. The eye is circular and the iris is yellowish-brown. A mature Copperhead is usually 1.2 metres long and the maximum recorded length is 1.83 metres.

The scales are smooth and are usually in 15 rows. Very rarely they may be in 13 or 17 rows. The ventrals number 140 to 160 and the anal plate is single. The 35 to 55 subcaudals are also single, so this snake can easily be distinguished from brown snakes and black snakes. On the head the frontal plate is much longer than that of the Mainland Tiger Snake, the length being almost twice the breadth.

The young are born alive and the usual litter is 18 to 20. They are usually much lighter in colour.

The Copperhead is inoffensive and rarely bites man. When angry it flattens its neck like the Mainland Tiger Snake, but is slower to strike and is relatively inaccurate. The average fang length is 3.3 mm and the longest length recorded is 4.5 mm.

The average venom yield is 26 mg and the maximum recorded is 85 mg. The venom is very toxic by world standards but less toxic than the more common Australian snakes. It causes paralysis and disturbances in blood clotting. It can also attack the muscles of the body.

Deaths or severe illnesses due to Copperheads are rare because the snake is reluctant to bite and usually bites inaccurately. However, it will bite when provoked. Some time ago a heavily built young man wearing thongs jumped off his tractor and landed on a Copperhead. The Copperhead inflicted several deep bites around his ankle. He was three hours from medical aid and when he arrived at hospital was critically ill, but responded well to tiger snake antivenom. This antivenom has been used for many years to treat Copperhead bites.

 Tiger snake antivenom may be used to treat bites by this snake.

 First Aid, see pages 1–2

# 8 Red-bellied Black Snake

*Pseudechis porphyriacus*

This beautiful snake rarely causes serious poisoning and does not deserve the attacks so often made upon it by humans. It is one of the best known Australian snakes and was once very common around Sydney. The Red-bellied or Common Black Snake is found in a patchy distribution down the eastern coast of Australia from the mountainous regions of Queensland through New South Wales to Victoria. It extends slightly into South Australia. This snake is not found in Western Australia, the Northern Territory or Tasmania.

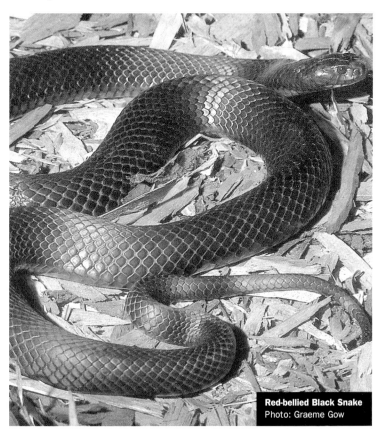

**Red-bellied Black Snake**
Photo: Graeme Gow

The Red-bellied Black Snake prefers well-watered areas such as swamps, rivers, creeks and lakes where there are lots of prey. It has a very large appetite and feeds on rats, mice, frogs, lizards and birds. It is a very good swimmer and catches fish and eels. Like the Copperhead, this snake is very prone to cannibalism. It hunts during the day. When alarmed it will try to escape into bushes or underground, usually successfully. If cornered it will hiss loudly, flatten its head and make bluffing strikes. Although this snake was greatly feared by the early settlers in New South Wales, it does not often cause illness in man.

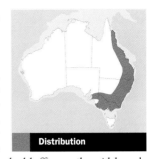

Distribution

The head of the Red-bellied Black Snake is small and not distinct from the neck. The body is a shiny purplish-black and the snout usually light grey. The sides are red or bright orange and it looks as if it has a red belly. However, the belly itself is usually dull red or pink. The underside of the tail is black. The colouring is almost the same wherever it is found, though northern specimens tend to have pale pink or light cream bellies. The average length is 1.25 metres and the maximum length recorded is 2.5 metres. This snake has 17 rows of body scales and 180 to 215 ventral scales with a divided anal plate. Subcaudals number 48 to 60. Sometimes all the subcaudals are single, but usually only the front ones are single and the remainder are divided.

The young are born alive and usually number from 12 to 20. Broods as large as 40 have been recorded. At birth the average length is 20 cm. Quite frequently the young are born in membranous sacs from which they escape within minutes of birth, though sometimes they may take up to an hour to escape.

The average venom yield upon milking is 37 mg and the maximum recorded is 94 mg. The venom is far less toxic than any of the other common dangerous Australian snakes. The subcutaneous $LD_{50}$ in 18 to 21 g mice is 2.5 mg/kg. It can cause paralysis, disturb blood clotting and attack the muscles of the body.

Although children have died from bites by this snake there are no confirmed deaths in adults.

Tiger snake antivenom is preferred to the larger volume black snake antivenom.

First Aid, see pages 1–2

# 9 Mulga *or* King Brown Snake

## *Pseudechis australis*

The name Mulga is preferable to King Brown because this snake is not a member of the brown snake genus (*Pseudonaja*) but belongs to the black snake genus (*Pseudechis*). This is very important because antivenom made against one genus will not usually neutralise the venom from the other.

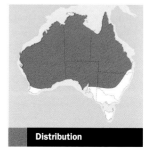

**Distribution**

The Mulga has a wide distribution in Australia but is not found in extremely dry areas or the extreme south of Western Australia, the south-eastern part of the continent or Tasmania. It feeds on rats, mice, lizards and birds and is particularly fond of eating other snakes. It often lives under logs or in rabbit holes. It is frequently active at night, especially in hot weather.

The Mulga is heavily built and its head is slightly distinct from the neck. The body is usually a uniform light brown, generally copper coloured or slightly reddish. Sometimes the body may be a dark olive-brown. Individual scales may occasionally be tipped with red. The belly is pinkish-cream, often with orange or pink blotching. The Mulga grows to be a very large snake. The average length is 1.5 metres and the maximum recorded is greater than 3 metres.

The mid-body scales are smooth and in 17 rows. There are 180 to 225 ventral scales and it is rare for the anal plate not to be paired. There are 50 to 75 subcaudal scales, and the front ones are usually single.

The Mulga snake lays eggs.

If angered, this snake may become very aggressive. Its body flattens and it strikes rapidly (sometimes repeatedly) and may actually chew the bitten area, thus increasing the amount of venom injected.

It produces more venom than other Australian snakes, with an average venom yield of 180 mg. John Cann in 1986 obtained a yield of 1350 mg from a single Mulga snake! This is a world record for venom production from any snake. The venom of the Mulga snake is less toxic than a number of other Australian snakes (subcutaneous LD$_{50}$ in 18 to 21 mg mice is 2.38 mg/kg). Although its venom is less potent, the large venom output makes it potentially extremely dangerous.

The venom appears to be different to that of other Australian snakes in that its major role is to attack the muscles of the body, causing paralysis by

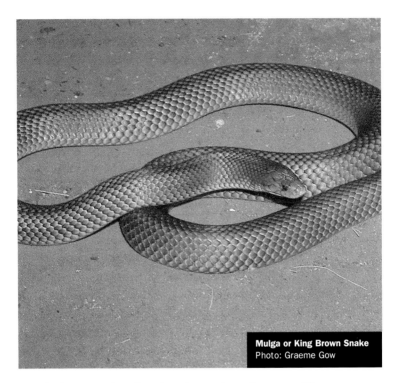

**Mulga or King Brown Snake**
Photo: Graeme Gow

muscle damage rather than directly attacking the nerves. The venom can also produce disturbances in blood clotting. Persons bitten by Mulga snakes often suffer from swelling and pain at the area of the bite. This is rare with other cases of snake bite in Australia and may be due to the large quantity of venom that is injected. Persons bitten by the Mulga may require large doses of black snake antivenom.

The False King Brown Snake, *Pailsus pailsei*, was recognised as a new species in October 1998. The two specimens described to date, which were both found near Mount Isa, have scalation and colour similar to the King Brown Snake, but their build resembles the brown snakes (Nos 3–6). Nothing is known yet about the extent of its distribution or its venom. In the meantime, if a person suffers a bite by this snake and requires antivenom, polyvalent antivenom should be used. A swab from the bite tested in a Snake Venom Detection Kit may throw light on the monovalent antivenom of choice.

 Black snake antivenom is the antivenom of choice.

 First Aid, see pages 1–2

# 10 Blue-bellied *or* Spotted Black Snake

## *Pseudechis guttatus*

This snake is found from south-eastern Queensland to the Hunter River district of New South Wales, where it is quite common. The Blue-bellied Black Snake prefers dry inland areas away from water. It is a nervous, shy snake and will try to avoid contact with humans.

It has a thick body and its head is slightly distinct from the neck. Its body is usually a very dark glossy black with or without cream spots, but sometimes it may be dark brown. The belly is a metallic blue-black occasionally with light yellow spots. The average length of a mature snake is 1.25 metres. The longest specimen ever found measured 2 metres. The body scales number 19 rows and there are 175 to 205 ventrals. There are 45 to 65 subcaudals; the rear third are divided, as is the anal plate.

The Blue-bellied Black Snake lays eggs.

When frightened this snake shows two characteristic features. It flattens its body out to a remarkable degree and emits a loud whistling sound. The length and the depth of its hiss is distinctive of this snake.

The average venom output of the Blue-bellied Black Snake is not known but its venom is the most poisonous in mice of any of the black snake venoms (subcutaneous $LD_{50}$ in 18 to 21 g mice is 2.13 mg/kg). Bites by this snake may cause severe local pain and tenderness of the lymph nodes near the wound. It should be considered a dangerous snake.

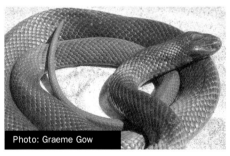

Photo: Graeme Gow

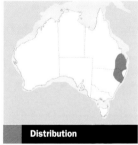

Distribution

 Tiger snake antivenom is the antivenom of choice.

 First Aid, see pages 1–2

# 11 Collett's Snake

## *Pseudechis colletti*

This rare but very attractive snake is limited to central Queensland. It can be found inland in non-swampy areas. It hunts by day and eats mainly lizards, small animals and other snakes.

Collett's Snake is solidly built with the head barely distinct from the neck. The body scales have individual colours which produce a characteristic appearance of spots and haphazard bands. The spots range from

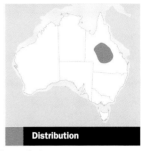

**Distribution**

brown to pink to light cream. The belly is either a light orange or creamy yellow. The average length of a mature snake is 1.25 metres and the maximum length recorded is 2 metres.

This snake has 19 rows of mid-body scales, the ventral scales number 215 to 235, and the anal plate is divided. The subcaudals number 50 to 70 and the scales in front are single.

Collett's Snake lays eggs, which usually number about 12.

Its venom has been shown to be as poisonous as that of the Mulga snake (*Pseudechis australis*) (No. 9) and mature specimens are considered to be dangerous to man.

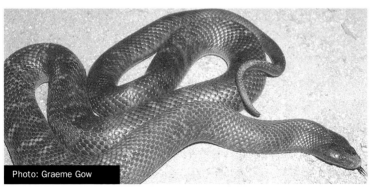

Photo: Graeme Gow

 Tiger snake antivenom should be used to treat victims of this snake.

 First Aid, see pages 1–2

# 12 | Death Adders

There are three main species of death adders in Australia. *Acanthophis praelongus* is found north of the Tropic of Capricorn. *A. pyrrhus* inhabits desert regions of central Australia and much of Western Australia except the extreme north and south of that state, and *A. antarcticus*, which is known as the Common Death Adder or 'Deaf Adder', is found in the remaining area of the distribution map. Death adders are not found in Tasmania, and it is very doubtful if they exist in Victoria. They are common throughout Papua New Guinea except in the Southern Highlands.

The Death Adder prefers undisturbed bushland where it can partially bury itself under leaves, sand or gravel. Often only a portion of its back and its worm-like tail are exposed. When resting it curls up so that its tail is immediately in front of its head. It twitches its tail to lure its prey. It eats frogs, birds, lizards, mice and young rats. This snake is generally only active at night. If discovered during the day, it usually makes no attempt to escape and is thus a serious danger to people walking near its hiding place. All

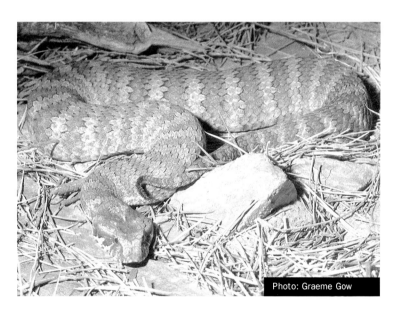

Photo: Graeme Gow

other Australian snakes, if they are awake, will generally retreat when they detect by vibration a person's approach. In many places snake bite at night is most likely to be caused by a Death Adder. However, in Victoria on hot summer evenings snake bite is most frequently caused by the Mainland Tiger Snake (No.1).

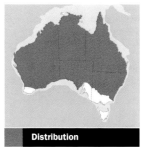

**Distribution**

The Death Adder looks different from other Australian snakes, resembling an overseas viper. It has a very broad (almost triangular) head, a thick neck and a short, fat body. The little tail ends in a small sting-like tip. The colour varies from one place to another, and striking variations may be found within a small area. It may be light brown, reddish-brown or even black. Distinct to indistinct bands of lighter or darker colours may cross the length of its body. The belly is yellowish or grey with pink or brown spots. The eye is quite small and the pupil is elliptical like a cat's eye. The average length of the snake is 0.65 metres and the maximum length recorded is 2.7 metres. The Common Death Adder has 21 to 23 rows of mid-body scales and the ventral scales number 110 to 130. The anal plate is undivided and sub-caudals, which are mostly undivided, number 40 to 55.

Death Adders are born alive and some 12 to 20 young are born in a litter each year.

There is evidence that the Death Adder only bites when it is touched, and many people have stood close to one which made no attempt to strike. When touched, it flattens its body and strikes with amazing speed, usually quite low to the ground. Bites usually occur to the foot, ankle or hand. The Death Adder seems never to waste its venom by striking an inanimate object. It has a very efficient biting apparatus as its fangs are amongst the longest, with an average length of 6.2 mm and a maximum recorded of 8.3 mm. The fangs are more mobile than any of the other Australian snakes.

The bone to which the fang is attached can rotate forward so that when the fang enters its victim it is at right angles and thus can penetrate more deeply.

Death Adders produce large quantities of venom with an average yield of 85 mg. The maximum yield reported is a stupendous 235 mg. The venom is extremely toxic, being the fifth most toxic Australian land snake venom. It is capable of causing a severe paralysis, and 50 per cent of its victims died in the days before an antivenom was available.

To avoid bites, wear protective footwear in snake country and always use a torch at night.

 **Death Adder antivenom is available.**

 **First Aid, see pages 1–2**

# 13 Taipan

## Oxyuranus scutellatus

The Taipan is the longest venomous snake in Australia. It has caused many human deaths and, before an antivenom became available in 1955, its bite was invariably fatal. It has very long fangs, produces large amounts of extremely potent venom, and is a particularly fast-moving snake.

Before 1977 it was thought that the Taipan lived in a wide area of northern Australia. However, what was called the Western Taipan is a different species, the Small-scaled or Fierce Snake (No. 14), and the Taipan is found only in the most northern parts of Australia extending down the coast to south of Brisbane. It has been found as far south as the Kimberleys in Western Australia and on a number of islands off the northern coast, including Melville Island. A close relative of the Taipan, *Oxyuranus canni*, is found in Papua New Guinea.

The Taipan usually hunts during the day. When the weather is extremely hot, it hunts in the evening. Its main diet is rats and mice, although it will eat small bandicoots or birds. Its fondness for rats and mice increases its chance of meeting humans because it will hunt them in farm buildings and garbage tips. The Taipan is not naturally aggressive and, when

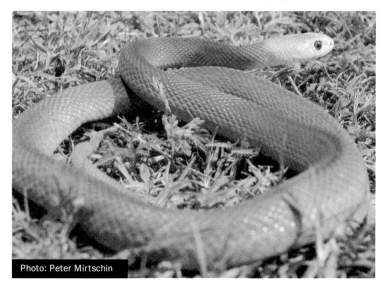

Photo: Peter Mirtschin

approached, will almost invariably attempt to escape. It shyness combined with the speed of its retreat is probably one reason it is considered a relatively rare snake. However, if the Taipan is cornered or attacked it becomes extremely aggressive and will strike a great speed, usually snapping three or four times in succession. There is very little chance of the victim escaping a bite. After a number of bites the snake, still snapping at intervals, may take hold of the victim.

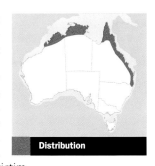

**Distribution**

The head is long and narrow and the Taipan has a remarkably delicate neck compared with its overall size. Adult Taipans are uniformly light or dark brown above with a creamy yellow belly that usually has reddish or pink spots towards the front. The belly has been described as having a beautiful mother of pearl bloom. The eye is quite large and the pupil is circular with an orange-yellow iris. The mouth is particularly large. The average length of the Taipan is 2.5 metres and the maximum recorded is 3.35 metres. The mid-body scales number 21 to 23 rows and the ventrals 220 to as many as 250. The anal plate is single and the 45 to 50 subcaudal scales are divided.

The Taipan lays eggs. Some 10 to 20 eggs are laid and they usually hatch after 12 weeks. The eggs are about 50 mm in length and are white at first but turn brownish-pink. When first hatched the snakes measure up to 56 cm in length.

The fangs of the Taipan are the longest of any of the venomous Australian snakes. The maximum length recorded is 13 mm. The Taipan is a copious producer of venom, with an average yield of 120 mg and a maximum yield of some 400 mg. The venom is third most toxic of any of the Australian snakes, with a subcutaneous $LD_{50}$ in 18 to 21 g mice of 0.099 mg/kg. It is extremely neurotoxic and may also cause severe changes in blood clotting.

Death from snake bite in Australia has now become rare due to improved patient care. However, the Taipan may still cause such severe poisoning that death may be almost inevitable. For example, in October 1979 a 4-year-old boy was attacked by a Taipan and received multiple bites to his groin and buttocks. The child was considered dead within 10 minutes, and at post-mortem large quantities of venom were found in tissue from the bitten area. It is indeed fortunate that this snake retreats when it senses human approach; usually the person is unaware that a Taipan has been in the vicinity.

 Taipan antivenom is used to treat victims.

 First Aid, see pages 1–2

# 14 Small-scaled *or* Fierce Snake

## *Oxyuranus microlepidotus*

L ive specimens of this snake were first collected and milked in 1975. The venom was found to be the most poisonous land snake venom yet discovered.

The Small-scaled Snake is found in isolated patches over a very large area (south-western Queensland, western New South Wales, and adjacent parts of the Northern Territory and South Australia). Most specimens have been collected from near the channel systems of Cooper Creek and the Diamantina River. In 1992 the known range of this snake was greatly extended when a number of specimens were found around Coober Pedy.

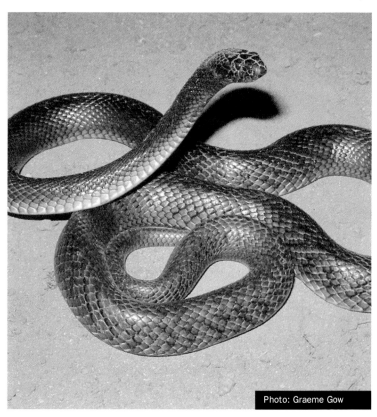

Photo: Graeme Gow

Little is known about the habits of this snake. In the ashy downs area of western Queensland it feeds upon the Long-haired Rat (*Rattus villossimus*) and often lives in the underground burrow network these rats excavate. When the rats become few the Small-scaled Snake may remain in the burrows for a long time without eating. In drought, when the ashy downs develop deep cracks, the snake shelters in their depths where it may survive long periods of intense heat without food or water.

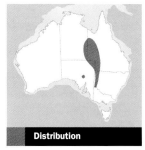

Distribution

In appearance it is very similar to the Taipan, and until recently it was known as the Western Taipan. The body is a deep brown above and the head is usually a glossy black. Some specimens have faint body banding, which is more marked near the tail. In summer the body colour fades greatly in all specimens. The belly is cream and its scales are tipped with brown at the side. The average length of specimens is 1.7 metres and the maximum size recorded is 2.7 metres. The scales are smooth and at mid-body are in 23 rows. The ventrals number 212 to 237 and the divided sub-caudals range from 54 to 66 in number. The anal plate is undivided.

The Small-scaled Snake lays some 9 to 12 eggs which incubate for about 66 days. When the young hatch they may measure more than 40 cm.

The description fierce is no more deserved by this species than any of the other dangerous Australian snakes. If sufficiently provoked it will certainly attack with unrestrained ferocity.

The average venom yield is 44 mg and the maximum yield recorded is 120 mg. This is sufficient to kill more than a quarter of a million mice! The venom of this snake is the most toxic land snake venom in the world with a subcutaneous $LD_{50}$ in mice of 0.025 mg/kg. A rat bitten by this snake would probably drop dead within a few seconds of the bite, as the venom is highly neurotoxic.

In the past, there has been little human contact with this snake because few people enter its habitat.

However now that it is represented in many collections of living reptiles a number of herpetologists have been bitten. One was bitten by a three-week old male specimen. He required urgent antivenom therapy and recovered. A pretty good effort for a baby snake—perhaps a world record!

 Taipan antivenom is used to treat victims.

 First Aid, see pages 1–2

## 15 Rough-scaled *or* Clarence River Snake

### *Tropidechis carinatus*

This is a highly nervous snake which by all accounts rarely hesitates to take the initiative in a fight. It is frequently found near the Clarence River in New South Wales, hence its name. Except for a region between Rockhampton and Tully, it lives in a large area along the eastern coast of Queensland.

The Rough-scaled Snake is usually found close to water, where it feeds mainly upon frogs and mice. It is normally active during the day but comes out in the evening when the weather is hot.

The snake is called rough-scaled because of its strongly keeled body scales. It has a large head which is distinct from its neck. The body is a greenish-brown, usually crossed with dark bands which fade on its sides. The belly is pale and usually has light green patches. The average length of

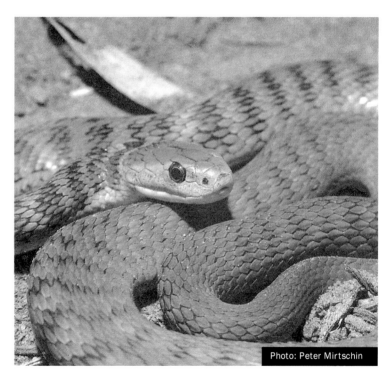

Photo: Peter Mirtschin

a mature specimen is 0.71 metres and the maximum length of this snake is 1.07 metres. The snake has 23 rows of body scales, the ventrals number 160 to 185 and the subcaudals 50 to 55. Both the anal plate the subcaudals are single.

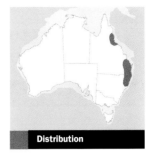

Distribution

A completely harmless aquatic snake is found in the same area as the Rough-scaled Snake. This is the Common Keel Back (*Tropidonophis mairii*), which is an inoffensive snake very unlikely to bite. It has 15 rows of body scales and its anal plate is divided. It is easy to tell apart from the Rough-scaled Snake because of the difference in scales.

The Rough-scaled Snake is highly strung and almost always retaliates if upset. When approached, it may adopt an aggressive pose and then make rapid strikes while it hisses frantically. In captivity it rarely becomes at all tame, unlike other snakes.

The average yield of venom from this snake is 14.5 mg and the subcutaneous $LD_{50}$ in 18 to 21 g mice is 1.36 mg/kg. The venom is very neurotoxic, causing disturbances in blood clotting and muscle damage. This snake has definitely caused deaths and is suspected of being responsible for a number of serious cases of snake bite in which the offending snake was unidentified.

A large number of snake collectors have been bitten by the Rough-scaled Snake which indicates that it is a snake which even the experts should avoid.

 **The venom is effectively neutralised by tiger snake antivenom.**

 **First Aid, see pages 1–2**

# 16 Eastern Small-eyed Snake

## *Rhinocephalus nigrescens*

**T**here is some controversy as to whether this snake is dangerous to man. It has a wide distribution over the ranges and coastal areas of eastern Australia from Victoria to Cape York.

The Small-eyed Snake is only active at night. It likes wooded areas, including rain forests, and lives under stones and fallen bark or in crevices in sandstone or rocky outcrops in the forest. Its main diet consists of small reptiles but occasionally it will eat frogs. This elegant looking snake has a slender body with a distinct neck. The body is usually a glistening black, but may be a greyish brown. The head is uniformly dark and the belly a light cream

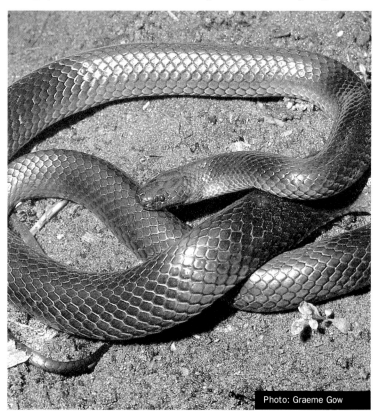

Photo: Graeme Gow

or pink, often with black spots. The average length is 0.5 metres and the maximum length is 1.2 metres. There are 15 rows of body scales and 165 to 210 ventrals. The 30 to 46 subcaudals are single, as is the anal plate.

The young are born free with litter sizes ranging from 2 to 5.

This snake is far from aggressive, but a number of humans have been bitten by it, the victims usually being snake handlers.

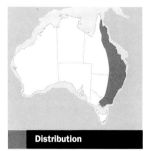

Distribution

The average venom yield is about 5 mg and it is of low toxicity in mice (subcutaneous $LD_{50}$ 2.67 mg/kg in 18 to 21 g mice). It is clearly established however, that its bites can be quite painful and they usually cause a severe headache. In 1965 a 20-year-old man died at Cairns Base Hospital 10 days after being bitten by a small specimen. The cause of death was kidney failure, thought to be a result of muscle damage probably due to the snake bite. Studies in monkeys show few toxic effects but some muscle damage may occur. Until further information is available about this snake, including its maximum venom output, it should be treated with caution.

 The Small-eyed Snake's venom is neutralised by tiger snake antivenom.

 First Aid, see pages 1–2

# 17 Broad-headed Snake

## *Hoplocephalus bungaroides*

This is a beautiful snake which is becoming rarer because it is a favourite collector's item. It is found from the outskirts of Sydney along rocky parts of the nearby coast, and as far as the neighbouring mountains.

The Broad-headed Snake is active by night and prefers dry rocky areas, such as the Hawkesbury sandstone region. It may be found hiding under large boulders or slabs of rock or in crevices. Its diet consists of geckoes, small skinks, mice, frogs and birds.

It is easily identified by its very broad head and striking colours. However, at first glance it may be confused with the harmless Diamond Python (*Morelia spilotes*). The back of the snake is jet black with irregular bands of bright yellow scales. A striking features is the yellow markings on its head and upper lip. The belly is usually dark grey and it may have yellow blotches. The average length of a mature specimen is 0.75 metres and

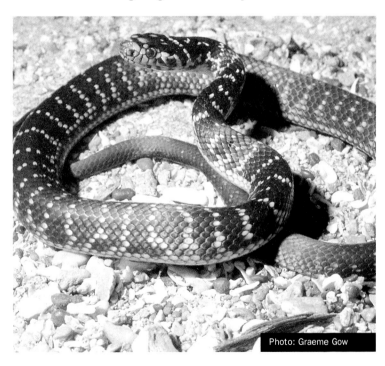

Photo: Graeme Gow

the maximum recorded is 1.52 metres. The scales are smooth and the mid-body scales are in 21 rows. The ventral scales number 200 to 230. The anal plate is single as are the 40 to 65 subcaudals. The young of the Broad-headed Snake are born free and litters range from 8 to 20.

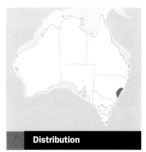

**Distribution**

When disturbed this snake becomes extremely agitated and may not hesitate to strike a number of times in rapid succession. The venom is neurotoxic and, although no human deaths have as yet been attributed to it, must be considered dangerous to man. Collectors who have been bitten by medium-sized specimens have suffered violent headaches, vomiting and partial loss of consciousness.

Tiger snake antivenom neutralises the venom of this snake.

 Tiger snake antivenom neutralises the venom of this snake.

 First Aid, see pages 1–2

# 18 Stephen's Banded Snake

*Hoplocephalus stephensi*

This is a handsome snake, some specimens of which may be unbanded. Its distribution ranges from the coastal ranges of Gosford, in New South Wales, to south-eastern Queensland.

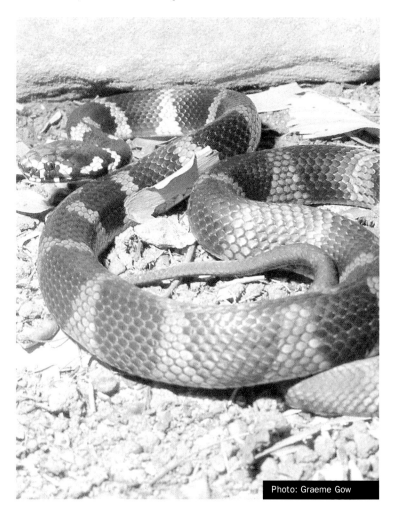

Photo: Graeme Gow

Stephen's Banded Snake likes living in trees and is often found under sheets of bark or in tree hollows, where it feeds on lizards, small mice and birds.

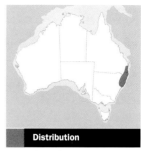

**Distribution**

In its usual banded form this snake's striking feature is the very broad dark bands along the length of its brown or yellowish body. Sometimes the bands are absent or may run along the body rather than round it. The broad head is spotted with black and the nape of the neck is usually a creamish-white with a dark collar at the back. The belly is light yellow covered with dark spots behind. The average length is 0.6 metres and the maximum length 1.0 metres. The body scales are in 21 rows and the ventrals number 220 to 250. The anal plate is single, as are the 50 to 70 subcaudals.

The young are born free and at birth may be as long as 17.5 cm.

Like other members of this genus, the snake is aggressive by nature even after mild provocation. When angry it raises its head high, bends its upper body into a tight S shape and strikes like an uncoiling spring.

The venom of Stephen's Banded Snake is highly toxic (subcutaneous $LD_{50}$ in 18 to 21 g mice is 1.36 mg/kg). A bite by a large specimen can cause a serious illness, especially in a child.

 Tiger snake antivenom neutralises the venom of this snake.

 First Aid, see pages 1–2

# 19 Pale-headed Snake

## *Hoplocephalus bitorquatus*

This is an attractive snake with a larger area of distribution than other members of the genus *Hoplocephalus*.

It is found from 80 kilometres north of Sydney to northern Queensland and its patchy distribution extends westwards to Dubbo and the Atherton Tableland.

It hunts by night and usually lives under the bark of trees, feeding upon small reptiles.

Its broad head is grey spotted with black, as are the lips. Behind the head is a cream or white band with or without dark spots. The body is uniform light grey or brown and the belly is a yellowish grey, sometimes with darker spots especially behind. The average length of this snake is 50 cm and the maximum recorded is 90 cm. There are 21 rows of body scales and the ventrals number 190 to 225. The 40 to 65 subcaudals are single as is the anal plate.

The Pale-headed Snake has a nervous temperament and does not hesitate to strike if threatened.

The venom is neurotoxic in action, and although the snake is not considered deadly it should be treated with great respect.

**Distribution**

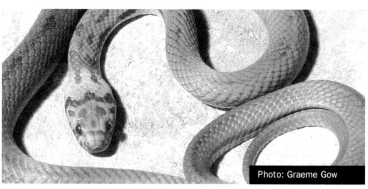

Photo: Graeme Gow

 Tiger snake antivenom neutralises the venom of this snake.

 First Aid, see pages 1–2

# 20 Sea snakes

## Family Hydrophiidae

Over 30 species of sea snakes are found in northern Australian waters. They are all venomous, but fortunately are shy and usually bite only when handled. Bites occur most frequently when the snakes have been caught in nets and are accidentally touched at night.

Two sea snakes with particularly wide distribution are the Yellow-bellied Sea Snake (*Pelamis platurus*) and *Hydrophis ornatus*. Both these species have been seen as far south as Tasmania. Sea snakes are often caught in the nets of prawning boats; in the Gulf of Carpentaria a minimum of one sea

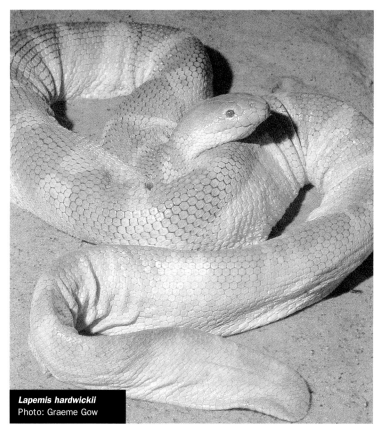

*Lapemis hardwickii*
Photo: Graeme Gow

snake is caught per hour of trawling. In this area the common species are *Lapemis hardwickii* and *Hydrophis elegans*.

Sea snakes are excellent swimmers and usually spend all their lives at sea. They frequently dive to considerable depths in search of fish and eels and may remain submerged for hours. A sea snake stores air in its right lung, which is very long and extends to the base of the tail. Some species like float-

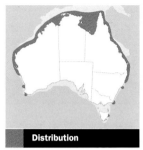

**Distribution**

ing on the surface and will quickly devour any inquisitive fish which has risen from the depths to investigate them. Sea snakes shed their skins as often as every two weeks, probably to prevent the build-up of marine growth. Sometimes hundreds of thousands of sea snakes may be found in a thickly knotted writhing mass several miles long. This behaviour was for many years incorrectly considered to be part of the breeding cycle.

Sea snakes are easily identified by their flattened, paddle-like tail and valvular nostrils. The Yellow-bellied Sea Snake has a clear division between its very dark black back and its yellow sides and belly. The tail is creamish-yellow with large dark blotches. The average length is less than 1 metre. The mid-body scales are in 49 to 67 rows and the ventral scales number 264 to 406. Scale counting on sea snakes can be very difficult for the amateur because of the large number of relatively tiny scales involved.

The Banded Sea Snake (*Laticauda colubrina*) comes ashore to lay up to 20 eggs, but the young of most other species are born alive at sea.

The fangs are small, fixed, and situated near the front of the mouth. Although only small quantities of venom are produced, it is in many cases extremely toxic. In humans the venom may cause death due to severe muscle damage. Sea snakes should never be picked up by the inexperienced, and great care should be taken when handling fishing nets in tropical waters, particularly at night.

The sea snake antivenom made in Australia against the venom of the Beaked Sea Snake (*Enhydrina schistosa*) combined with tiger snake antivenom has been found to neutralise all the important sea snake venoms. There is evidence that tiger snake antivenom alone is highly effective in neutralising the venom of most sea snakes.

 **Sea snake antivenom is used to treat bites by these snakes. If this is not available, tiger snake antivenom may be used.**

 First Aid, see pages 1–2

# Ants, Bees, and Wasps

# 21 Stinging ants

**A**ustralia has a number of species of highly aggressive ants. Everywhere there are stinging ants and some of them have venom which, as well as producing an immediately painful sting, can cause the development of an allergy which may be fatal in humans.

The most dangerous ants are the Jumper Ant (*Myrmecia pilosula*) and Bull Ant (*Myrmecia pyriformis*), of which there are a number of types found in the south and south-west of the country in all kinds of environments. They are amongst the most primitive ants in the world. Jumper and Bull Ants are highly aggressive and show little fear when humans trespass on their territory. They have powerful front jaws or mandibles with which they grasp their victims. When the skin is firmly held by the mandibles, the ant will curl up its body and thrust a long, sharp barbless sting into the victim. The sting is situated on the tail of the ant and it can enter the skin a number of times in quick succession, injecting more venom each time. Jumper Ants, or Jack Jumpers as they are sometimes called, have the additional advantage of being able to jump a few centimetres at a time.

Another ant which is important, particularly in the more central parts of Australia, is the Green-head Ant (*Rhytidopenera metallica*). The Green-head Ant tends to be a problem around houses in sub-tropical areas because it likes suburban lawns.

The venom of ants is as complex as the venom of a wasp (Nos. 23–25). Ant stings cause instantaneous burning pain which will increase over 5 minutes and settle to a throbbing discomfort which may last some hours. There is usually some swelling in the stung area. Sometimes multiple stings may be inflicted, particularly on young children, and they may need hospital treatment for pain and shock.

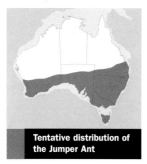

**Tentative distribution of the Jumper Ant**

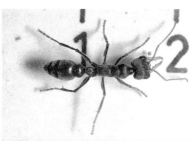

**Jumper Ant (scale in cm)**     Photo: Vern Draffin

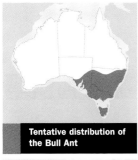
**Tentative distribution of the Bull Ant**

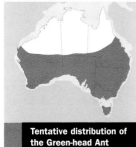
**Tentative distribution of the Green-head Ant**

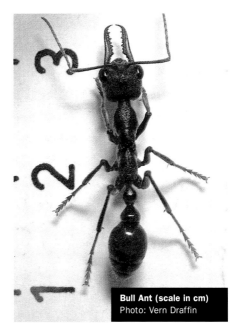
**Bull Ant (scale in cm)**
Photo: Vern Draffin

The development of an allergy to ant venom is the most important medical aspect of the sting. After the first sting the reaction is as described above. A second sting some time later may produce a similar degree of pain, but otherwise the reaction will be more severe. There may be severe local swelling, a generalised rash, difficulty in breathing or collapse. If there is any definite increase in the victim's reaction he or she should seek medical aid. If a high degree of allergy develops, patients should be given access to injectible adrenaline at all times in case of an emergency. The Australian Venom Research Unit is seeking funding to complete work on purified venom extracts for both the testing of patients and immunotherapy to diminish this dangerous allergy. (See also notes on Honey Bee venom allergy, page 56.)

In recent years the incidence of allergy to ants, in particular Jumper and Bull Ants, appears to have increased. This may be due to the numbers of houses which are built on large blocks of land and to the virtual elimination of the ant's natural enemy, the Short-beaked Echidna, also called the Spiny Anteater. The shooting of Echidnas, their slaughter on the roads, and the erection of stout fences against the survivors have all increased the risk of ant stings.

 Note for Doctor: see 'Venom Allergy and Anaphylaxis', page 8

 First Aid, see page 3

# 22 Honey Bee

## *Apis mellifera*

**B**ees, both the native species and the European Honey Bee, are found all over Australia, wherever there is pollen.

Stings by native bees only occasionally need medical attention, but major problems are caused by stings from the Honey Bee. Bee stings are barbed, unlike ant and wasp stings, so once the sting has been driven into the victim it is usually not possible for the bee to remove it. It is anchored firmly in the

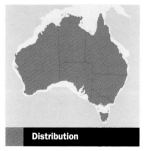

**Distribution**

skin and, when the bee swivels around, the sting and its associated venom gland is torn out and left behind. As a result the bee dies because of the damage to its abdomen, and the venom gland, which is still attached to the sting, continues its automatic pumping action and injects more venom into the victim.

Bee venom is very complicated. As well as giving immediate pain it is very likely to cause an allergy in the victim. There may be as many as 90 000 Australians who could have severe reactions (which might even be life-threatening) if they received another bee sting. Bee venom allergy is commonest amongst the families of those who keep bees either as a livelihood or a hobby, but the only reason that beekeepers' families are more likely to suffer from this allergy is that they are more likely to be in contact with bees than other members of the population. Beekeepers themselves very frequently develop a remarkable immunity to stings and often barely notice a veritable battery of them.

The development of bee venom allergy follows a similar pattern to the development of ant venom allergy (No. 21). Because of extensive research overseas and in Australia, doctors are in a much better position to investigate and treat persons allergic to bee venom than they were some years ago. Anyone suffering a more severe local reaction to a second or subsequent bee sting or any significant general reaction after a bee sting should seek medical advice as soon as possible.

For many years patients were treated with whole body extracts over a period of months. This process, which was called desensitisation or immunotherapy, is now known to work only if minute amounts of pure Honey Bee venom are employed. Bee venom specially prepared for immunotherapy is available in Australia as a pharmaceutical benefit.

Treatment must be given with the greatest care and is generally best supervised at least initially by an allergist, unless the particular doctor has considerable experience in such therapy.

Bee stings can often be avoided by not wearing bright clothes, particularly on sunny days when bees are active, and not using perfumes which may attract bees. Finally, especially where there are children, it is important that clover, which attracts bees, be selectively sprayed on suburban lawns.

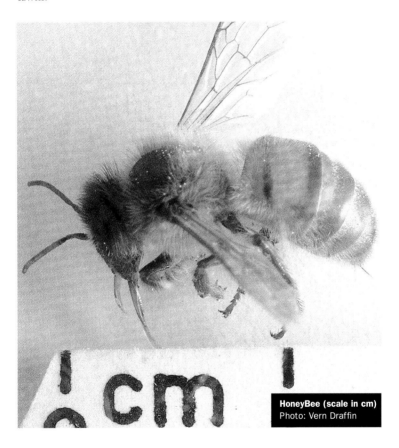

**HoneyBee (scale in cm)**
Photo: Vern Draffin

 **Note for Doctor: see 'Venom Allergy and Anaphylaxis', page 8**

 **First aid: see page 3**
**Scrape or pull the sting and attached venom sac off as fast as possible.**
**Speed is the essence!**

# 23 Paper Wasps

## *Polistes humilis, Polistes tasmaniensis*

**N**ative paper wasps (*Polistes humilis* and *Polistes tasmaniensis*) are found all over the country in forests or bush. They build large communal colonies on low-hanging foliage where their nests may be knocked by a passer-by. Like ants, wasps have barbless stings, so multiple stings can be inflicted and the wasp is usually not damaged. An allergy to wasp venom can be as serious as an allergy to bee venom, but it is not as common because there are fewer wasps.

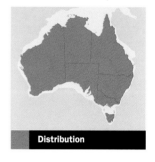

**Distribution**

 Note for Doctor: see 'Venom Allergy and Anaphyllaxis', page 8

 First Aid, see page 3

# 24 Blue Ant

## *Diamma bicolor*

One common wasp is usually not recognised as one. This is the 'Blue Ant' (*Diamma bicolor*), a wingless female wasp. It has a metallic blue body nearly 3 cm long and is often dug up by suburban gardeners. It has a large sting which can inflict an injury as severe or greater than a bee sting, but fortunately allergy is uncommon because it is most unusual for a person to receive more than one sting. The male wasp is rarely seen; he is much smaller and has black wings.

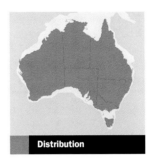

Distribution

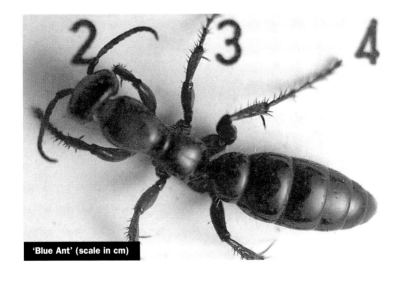

'Blue Ant' (scale in cm)

 **Note for Doctor:** see 'Venom Allergy and Anaphyllaxis', page 8

 First Aid, see page 3

# 25 European and English Wasps

*Vespula vulgaris and Vespula germanicus*

Imported wasps such as the English Wasp (*Vespula vulgaris*) and the European Wasp (*Vespula germanicus*) have spread through many suburban gardens, especially in Melbourne. They establish large nests usually at ground level, and will attack anyone who disturbs them. The nests should be promptly destroyed; advice on the best method can be obtained from local councils or State Agriculture Departments. Some Departments have excellent leaflets on the problem.

These wasps are becoming a significant menace. They will eat anything from meat to tomato sauce, and may aggressively disrupt a pleasant Sunday barbecue. Drinks should never be drunk directly from a container outdoors, because an unnoticed wasp may be inside; always use a straw.

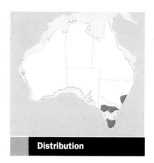

Distribution

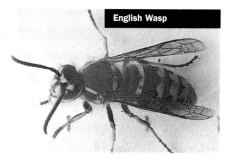

English Wasp

First Aid, see page 3

# Spiders and Ticks

## Introduction

The Sydney Funnel-web spider was not proved to be dangerous to man until 1927, and it is quite possible that a number of relatively common spiders of widespread distribution in Australia may, in time, prove to be quite important hazards to health. The major problem in deciding which creatures are dangerous and which are not is the common failure to identify the exact species of spider responsible for a bite which has led to serious illness. Until more is discovered about Australian spiders it is wise to treat all spiders with caution and to wear gloves when gardening. Anyone bitten by a spider should try to catch or identify the spider in case the bite causes a serious illness.

Museum experts can often identify even a mangled spider from its 'hard parts'. It is therfore helpful to preserve any intact spider or its remains in methylated spirits in case precise identification is warranted later. It is kind to freeze the live spider first to minimise its suffering.

# 26 White-tailed Spider

## *Lampona cylindrata*

**S**pecies of *Lampona* are found in most parts of Australia, often roaming about inside houses. The White-tailed Spider has a dark grey cylindrical body about 15 mm in length, and both sexes usually have a white strike or spot just above the spinnerets at the end of the abdomen. Bites by this spider can definitely cause skin damage, and sometimes ulcers at least one centimetre in diameter.

The White-tailed Spider is under suspicion as a cause of far more serious skin damage. Time will tell.

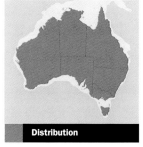

**Distribution**

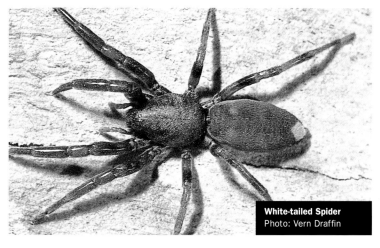

**White-tailed Spider**
Photo: Vern Draffin

**First aid:** No first aid is recommended following bites by the White-tailed Spider.
**Note for the Doctor:** see 'Necrotising Arachnidism' page 9.

# 27 Red-back Spider

*Latrodectus hasselti*

**H**undreds of people are bitten by female Red-backs every year. Its close relative, the Black Widow spider, is probably the most common cause of serious spider bites overseas. An almost identical spider, the Katipo, is the only venomous creature (except for stinging insects) found in New Zealand. In 1987 the Brown Widow Spider was found in Brisbane. This is not considered highly dangerous to humans, but nonetheless it could make young children quite ill. Its venom would be neutralised by Red-back antivenom.

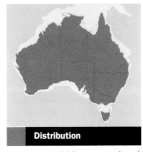

**Distribution**

The Red-back is found in all parts of Australia except in the hottest deserts and on the coldest mountains. It is the *only* highly dangerous spider with an Australia-wide distribution. Red-backs are very common in the summer.

Mature females spin untidy webs, usually in some quiet dark area under houses, at the backs of garages, amongst garden or industrial rubbish and, of course, in outside toilets. The web consists of 3 separate parts: a snare, trap threads and a retreat. The snare is a central tangled mass of web from which very sticky trap threads radiate. The tubular retreat usually extends into some suitable crevice where the spider hides during the day.

The female Red-back has a spherical satin-black abdomen with an orange-red stripe. The abdomen is usually about 1 cm in diameter. Eight long delicate legs arise from the tiny front segment of the body. The male is only about one-third the size of the female and is considered harmless to humans because his fangs are so small. It is usually easy to identify a female Red-back, although sometimes her stripe may be orange, pink, or even light grey.

After mating, the female spins up to 8 round balls of web for her eggs. Some of these may contain more than 500 eggs. If the weather is warm, the spiderlings hatch after about 2 weeks and will moult several times as they grow before they reach full size. Like many spiders, the young are very cannibalistic and only a few reach maturity.

Unlike the Sydney Funnel-web Spider, the Red-back is rarely aggressive and if molested will usually fall to the ground, curl up and feign death. If disturbed while guarding her eggs or cornered, she will bite the intruder

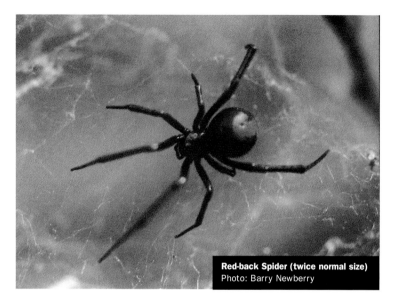

**Red-back Spider (twice normal size)**
Photo: Barry Newberry

with her minute but effective fangs. Most bites occur when the spider is trapped against the skin e.g. when old clothing containing the spider is put on or rubbish from a garage corner is picked up without inspection. More bites occur on the hands and feet than the rest of the body combined.

Although this spider injects only a tiny amount of venom it can cause serious illness, and deaths used to occur before an antivenom became available in 1956. The action of its venom is unique. It can attack all the nerves of the body and in severe cases causes a paralysis which may lead to death. At first the bite is only as painful as a minor insect sting. After a few minutes the pain becomes intense and spreads to other parts of the body. A special feature only seen with Red-back spider bites is that, when the joint pains and patches of sweating develop, they may move from one part of the body to another. The patients are particularly miserable and rarely sleep properly.

Fortunately, the serious effects of the venom take hours or even days to develop and there is plenty of time for treatment with antivenom. A unique finding is that the antivenom can be effective days or weeks after the bite has occurred.

*Remember*, most bites can be avoided. Keep your eyes open when going into those quiet little corners where the Red-back Spider makes its home. Its bright red stripe is nature's warning!

 Red-back Spider antivenom is available to treat bites.

 First Aid, see page 3

# 28 Sydney Funnel-web Spider

## Atrax robustus

The male Sydney Funnel-web Spider is one of the most dangerous in the world. Children have died less than 2 hours after being bitten. No serious illness has occurred after bites by the female.

The Sydney Funnel-web is believed to be limited to within 160 kilometres from the centre of Sydney. A number of other dangerous Funnel-web spiders are found in both Queensland and New South Wales (see No. 29). To date no illnesses have been reported following the rare bites by the species found in other states.

The Sydney Funnel-web constructs its own burrow, which may be over a foot deep, or uses a suitable crevice in rocks or around house foundations. Sometimes funnel-webs may be found in colonies of over a hundred. The webs are white and often tubular rather than funnel-like, with trip lines running out to surrounding rocks and debris. Only funnel-web spiders make such trip lines.

The spiders may take several years to reach maturity and the female may live for perhaps 8 years or longer. When mature, the males leave their webs and lead a homeless existence.

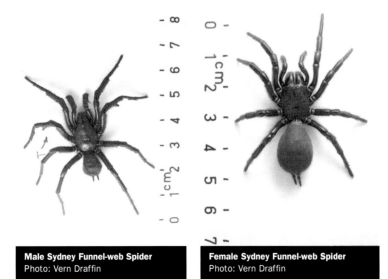

**Male Sydney Funnel-web Spider**
Photo: Vern Draffin

**Female Sydney Funnel-web Spider**
Photo: Vern Draffin

They tend to roam and often enter houses, particularly during the summer after a heavy downpour of rain. They mate with a female for only one season, and if not killed shortly after mating usually die within a few months.

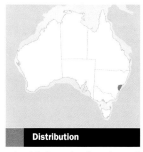

**Distribution**

This spider is one of Australia's largest and most easily identified. The paired spinnerets at the end of the abdomen are particularly long, much longer than those of other large dark spiders. The male is of a more delicate build than the female and has two features which help identification. One is a little spur half way along its second leg on each side and the other is finely pointed feelers for transferring sperm to the female.

Both sexes are very aggressive and when approached will usually rear up into a ready-to-strike position. (Folklore has it that their massive fangs can penetrate a child's finger nail.) However, most people bitten by them are not injected with sufficient venom to cause any illness. Often it falls off the tips of the spider's fangs as it makes a preliminary downward thrust. People bitten by the female spider may, at the most, suffer pain around the bitten area.

The venom of the male spider is five times more toxic than the female. Humans and monkeys appear to have a special susceptibility to the venom. For example, rabbits can be given very large doses of the venom with no apparent effect, but a small dose injected into a monkey produces the terrifying symptoms seen in some humans. In all human cases where the victim has died and in which the spider involved has been positively identified, it has been a male spider.

The venom contains a low molecular weight toxin called robustoxin which attacks the nerves of the body, causing thousands of electrical impulses to be fired down them. The muscles of the body twitch and there is a profuse flow of perspiration, tears and saliva. The venom also causes changes to blood vessels which can lead to shock and coma due to brain damage. All the evidence suggests that the effects wear off after a few hours. Provided the victim reaches hospital before serious illness has developed, he or she has an excellent chance of recovery. No deaths have occurred since an antivenom for the Sydney Funnel-web spider became available in 1980. Over a hundred patients have received it and it has so far proven reaction-free.

 Sydney Funnel-web Spider antivenom is available.

 First Aid, see page 3

# 29 Northern Tree-dwelling Funnel-web Spider

## *Hadronyche formidabilis*

In 1986 Dr Michael Gray of the Australian Museum reclassified this spider so that it left the genus *Atrax* to join the genus *Hadronyche*, as have all but three of the other thirty-two former members of *Atrax*. The distribution of these spiders and other details can be found in the book edited by Covacevich *et al.* listed under 'Further Reading' on page 127. Without doubt *H. formidabilis*, the Northern Tree-dwelling

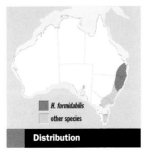

H. formidabilis

other species

**Distribution**

Funnel-web Spider, is a most dangerous member of this genus. Other members of genus *Hadronyche* which have caused serious illness are the Towoomba or Darling Downs Funnel-web Spider, *H. infensa* (Queensland), the Blue Mountains Funnel-web Spider, *H. versuta* and the Southern Tree-dwelling or Paper-bark Funnel-web Spider, *H. cerberea*. To date, all the patients have responded well to the antivenom made against *A. robustus* venom.

Specimens of the Northern Tree-dwelling Funnel-web Spider have been found from northern New South Wales to southern Queensland. It usually inhabits heavily timbered areas which are rarely entered by humans. Although it is sometimes known as the Tree-dwelling Funnel-web Spider, it does not always live above ground. In recent years some specimens have been found in fallen logs or in excavated tunnels. Timber cutters in the rain forests of northern New South Wales should take special care when cutting up recently felled trees. A Northern Funnel-web spider may make her nest in a hole as high as 18 metres from the base of the tree.

This is the largest of the funnel-web spiders and the female spider is truly formidable. The male is seen even less often than the female and may be distinguished from the male Sydney Funnel-web spider by the fact that the small spike on the second leg is blunt whereas in the Sydney Funnel-web it is quite pointed. Another difference between the two species is that in the Northern Funnel-web (and you need a microscope to see this) the intermediate teeth occupy the full length of the fang groove.

Little is known about the venom from either male of female specimens of this funnel-web spider. A disturbing finding was made when the venom of the large female pictured below, was examined. This spider, which was captured on Black Mountain, near Armidale, produced copious amounts of

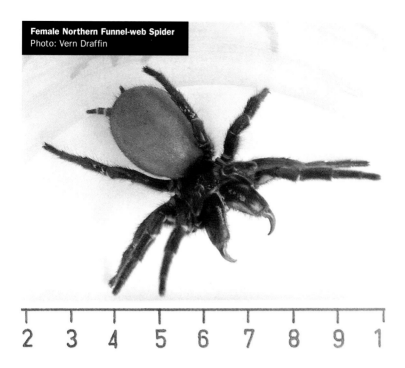

**Female Northern Funnel-web Spider**
Photo: Vern Draffin

2 3 4 5 6 7 8 9 1

venom at least as potent as male Sydney Funnel-web Spider venom. This suggests it is as dangerous as it looks!

The first recorded human victim of the Northern Funnel-web Spider was a timber cutter, a heavily built man. Several hours after being bitten by the spider he developed intense vomiting, perspiration and violent pains in the limbs. He became delirious and claimed someone was spraying him with something. He remained semi-comatose for a number of hours and took several days to recover fully. As the human population increases this spider will probably become a greater public health problem.

The antivenom developed against the venom of the Sydney Funnel-web effectively neutralises the venom of the Northern Tree-dwelling Funnel-web Spider. It has saved the life of at least one victim of this spider. The spider involved was a male.

 Sydney Funnel-web Spider antivenom is suitable to treat the bites of all *Hadronyche* spiders

 First Aid, see page 3

# 30 Wolf spiders

## Genus *Lycosa*

**T**here are literally dozens of species of wolf spiders in Australia and new species are regularly being found. They are very common in suburban gardens.

They are small to medium-sized spiders, drab coloured but often strikingly patterned in black and shades of grey, brown or orange. Their hunting ground is in foliage and at the edge of water. They are often seen scuttling away, sometimes carrying their egg sacs, when lawn edges are being trimmed. Some of them make shallow burrows, placing debris around the entrance.

Although when approached this spider may not adopt an aggressive stance like the Sydney Funnel-web Spider, it is possible that it inflicts bites when it is brought into direct contact with the skin of gardeners. Overseas species of *Lycosa* are known to produce ulcers of the skin near the bite site and may even cause death.

Some Australians have developed small punched-out areas of skin loss following bites in the garden by an unidentified creature. The wolf spider is a suspect and it may even cause far more serious injuries. For example, a

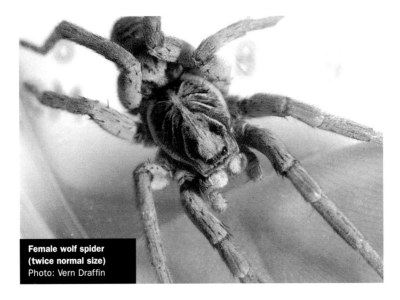

**Female wolf spider (twice normal size)**
Photo: Vern Draffin

young woman suffered patchy gangrenous changes to her left hand and life-threatening swellings of the arm and neck following a possible bite by a wolf spider, and severe kidney damage has developed in some patients several days after a definite bite by this spider. Even domestic animals are not safe, and it has been recorded that a fully grown Labrador died a few hours after a bite by *Lycosa godeffroyi*.

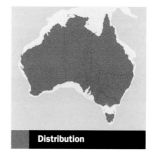

**Distribution**

 First aid: No first aid is recommended following bites by wolf spiders.
Note for the Doctor: see 'Necrotising Arachnidism' page 9.

# 31 Mouse Spider

## Missulena occatoria

**S**tudies of the venom of the female Mouse Spider suggests that it may be as potentially dangerous as the male Sydney Funnel-web Spider. No studies have been done on the venom of the male spider, but the female is a copious venom producer and her venom appears extremely poisonous.

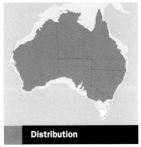

**Distribution**

The Mouse Spider is one of the trap-door spiders. It is dark, often black and thick-set in appearance. In the male the fangs and the neighbouring head parts are bright red. It makes vertical burrows lined with coarse silk, with two oval doors at the entrance. The females and immature spiders often remain hidden in the burrows.

It is an aggressive spider which adopts an attacking posture when approached or disturbed. Its large fangs and high venom output suggest that it may prove to be extremely dangerous to humans.

An infant in Queensland who was bitten by a male of another species of Mouse Spider (*Missulena bradleyi*) developed a severe illness. She did not respond to any therapy and was given funnel-web antivenom because of the similarity of this spider's venom to funnel-web venom. She improved rapidly and fully recovered. This case drew attention to the potential danger that Mouse Spiders present on the Australian mainland.

Other smaller species of the Mouse Spider genus have not been studied but their venom output seems to be quite low.

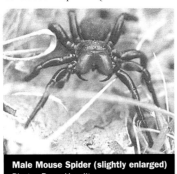

**Male Mouse Spider (slightly enlarged)**
Photo: Ross Hamilton

First aid: Pressure–immobilisation should be used in the case of a child bitten by a Mouse Spider. If an illness develops seek medical advice, taking the spider with you if possible.

# 32 Black House Spider *or* Window Spider

## *Baduma insignis*

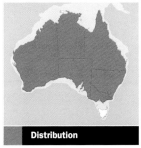

**Distribution**

The Black House Spider is a very common household spider which can usually be found in an untidy funnel-like web in the corners of windows in garages or in crevices in trees. The old webs look dense, thick and grey and the spider can often be seen at night repairing or adding to its web. It is a brownish-black or grey spider, the body of which usually does not grow longer than 1.5 cm.

Persons bitten by this spider have complained of severe pain around the area of the bite and have occasionally suffered generalised sweating, weakness and sometimes vomiting. The Black House Spider is known to cause significant local reactions, and the venom is currently being studied at the Australian Venom Research Unit.

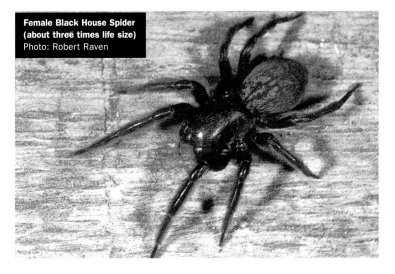

**Female Black House Spider
(about three times life size)**
Photo: Robert Raven

First aid: No first aid is recommended for bites of these spiders. If an illness develops seek medical advice, taking the spider with you if possible.
Note for the Doctor: see 'Necrotising Arachnidism' page 9.

# 33 Fiddleback Spider

## *Loxosceles rufescens*

In 1974 a specimen of the Fiddleback Spider was found in a western suburb of Adelaide. The discovery of a member of this family in Australia gave cause for concern, because species of this spider (which have common names such as Fiddleback, Violin or Brown Recluse) occasionally cause severe and even fatal illnesses in humans in overseas countries. Bites by these spiders, e.g. the American Brown Recluse (*Loxoscles reclusa*),

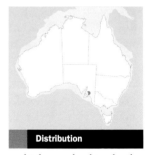

**Distribution**

may produce skin ulcers and/or kidney damage which may lead to death.

Research has shown that the Australian Fiddleback spider is found not only in the suburbs of Adelaide but also in a number of country areas of South Australia. Indeed, studies by Dr. Southcott show that the species has been present in museum collections for some 60 years.

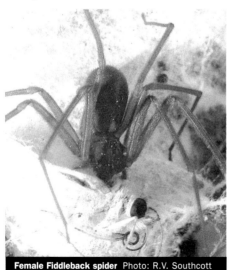

**Female Fiddleback spider** Photo: R.V. Southcott

It may be that man has little to fear from this spider. It is shy and retiring, usually only active at night. However, it is sensible to treat it, like all other spiders, with great caution. Each year a number of people who are bitten in or around their homes develop moderately severe illnesses which cannot be attributed to a specific creature because the offending animal has not been identified.

**First aid: No special first aid is recommended for Fiddleback Spider bites.**

74

# 34 Australian Paralysis Tick

## *Ixodes holocyclus*

The Australian Paralysis Tick has a poison in its saliva which can produce a progressive and sometimes even fatal paralysis in both humans and domestic animals. It can also cause a severe allergy in some people.

This tick is found along the coastal side of Australia's mountains from Queensland down to the rain forests of eastern Victoria. Whereas the Cattle Tick (*Boophilus microplus*) is a one-host species, the Paralysis

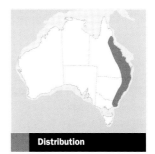

Distribution

Tick will attach itself to any warm-blooded animal which brushes the foliage on which it has been patiently waiting. The tick's commonest host is the bandicoot, but many other animals have suffered infestation. Dogs,

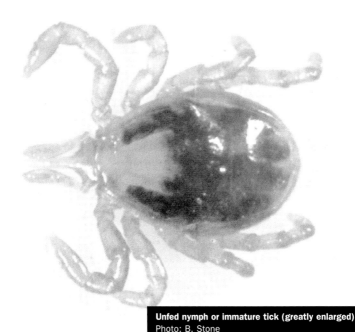

**Unfed nymph or immature tick (greatly enlarged)**
Photo: B. Stone

in particular, are often host to the tick, and in practice heavily infested dogs are used as a source of tick antivenom.

The life cycle of the tick is quite complicated, and during each of the three stages of the cycle the female must attach herself to a warm-blooded animal for a meal of blood. The male does not need to drink blood during the third stage. In some places

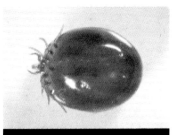

**Engorged nymph (greatly enlarged)**
Photo: B. Stone

thousands of ticks may climb plants and wait for a host to pass by. The immature form of the tick is the size of a pin's head. When it touches the skin of the host, its well-designed mouth pieces start engorging blood as it becomes partially buried in the skin. In four days the tick may have increased its size by up to 400 times and taken on the appearance of a small blood blister. At this stage the tick will usually extricate herself (it is usually a female) and drop off the host to digest its meal.

Families which picnic in tick-infested areas may not know that, as they leave for home, they have taken with them a number of tiny ticks. The ticks will hide themselves above the hairline of the scalp or in any of the skin creases of the body; they have even been known to attach themselves to the ear drum.

Over the next four days, as the tick enlarges, its toxin may attack the host. By the fifth day the victim may be showing signs of paralysis and, unless the doctor knows that the family has recently been into tick country, the illness may be confused with some other disease such as infantile paralysis. Indeed, sometimes ticks have not been recognised and have been covered by a bandage which has been left on until the child has died. Deaths due to tick poisoning are rare, however; some 20 people have died this century in New South Wales from this cause. Tick antitoxin is available.

*Remember*, after being in tick country *all* members of the family and any pets should be checked daily for six days in case ticks have been carried home.

 Tick antitoxin is available.

 First Aid, see page 3

# Other land creatures

# 35 Centipedes

## Order Scolopendromorpha

**C**entipedes are found throughout Australia in all environments, but most bites occur in suburban gardens.

Centipedes have a pair of fangs with which the larger specimens can inflict painful bites and introduce a quantity of usually innocuous venom. The appendage at the tail does not inject venom. They have not been reported to have killed anyone in Australia and there is only one death that

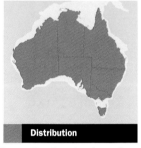

**Distribution**

has ever been attributed to them, when a child on a Pacific island was bitten on the skull by a large centipede. The largest centipedes of northern Australia, however, can produce very painful bites, and the victim may be uncomfortable for days.

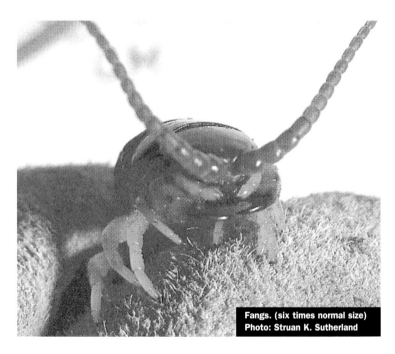

**Fangs. (six times normal size)**
**Photo: Struan K. Sutherland**

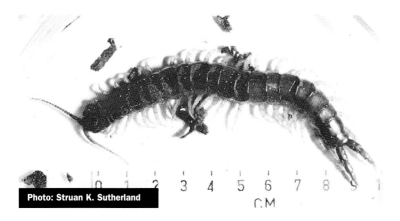

In 1976 in suburban Melbourne a healthy young man was bitten on the thumb by a moderate-sized centipede. He ignored the bite but some 10 minutes later collapsed and seemed to be pulseless and to have stopped breathing. By the time he got to hospital he had fully recovered. Centipedes should be treated with respect.

 **First aid: No specific first aid is recommended. If the pain persists or a general illness develops, then medical care may be required.**

# 36 Platypus

## Ornithorhynchus anatinus

There is no creature in the world even remotely like the Platypus. It is a duck-billed furry mammal which lays eggs. Although some years ago the Platypus population had declined due to hunting, it is increasing again.

Platypuses are completely protected. They are quite abundant in the streams and rivers of eastern Australia, Tasmania, and the south-east of South Australia. They are

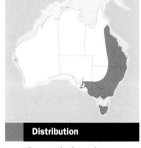

**Distribution**

found in any water that is free from pollution. They inhabit the warm coastal rivers and the icy mountain streams at altitudes as high as 1500 metres.

Except when they are mating, Platypuses tend to live alone. At dawn and dusk they can be found diving in the beds of rivers looking for worms and yabbies. They have a voracious appetite and when in captivity it is often difficult to supply them with enough food.

The Platypus excavates, in the river bank, a winding burrow with a number of side branches where it hides during the day. The burrow is semi-circular in cross-section and usually 5 to 10 metres long, but may be up to 30 metres in length. The breeding season is usually in July or August in the

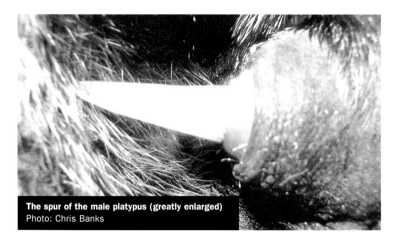

**The spur of the male platypus (greatly enlarged)**
Photo: Chris Banks

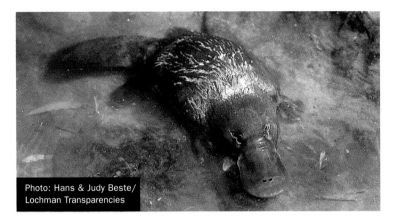

Photo: Hans & Judy Beste/
Lochman Transparencies

northern parts of Australia, but in the cooler southern parts breeding occurs in October. The female digs a breeding burrow and builds a nest at the extreme end, which is then blocked with earth while she is laying and incubating the eggs. From 1 to 3 eggs are laid and they are stuck together.

A mature male Platypus may be 60 cm long and weigh 2.4 kg. The female grows to about two-thirds the size of the male. The male has a venomous spur on the inside of each rear leg. These paired spurs are stout but sharp, and each is connected to a whitish kidney-shaped venom gland. The size of the venom gland varies, being largest during the breeding season. Scientists are undecided as to what the male platypus uses his spurs for. They may be a defence against other males, or they may be used to subdue the female. The Platypus stings by driving his hind legs towards one another, so that the victim's body is impaled between them and the venomous spurs penetrate the skin. Victims sometimes have difficulty in forcing the animal's legs apart to free themselves.

The venom contains a number of enzymes which cause local pain and tissue damage. In experimental animals the venom has produced death by respiratory failure and paralysis. A person stung by a Platypus may suffer extreme pain and swelling at the site of the wound for days. When the leg is stung there is a tendency for the swelling to redevelop if the patient has not rested long enough. A severe sting may require immobilisation for a number of days. There have been no deaths due to Platypus stings in Australia, and now that the creature is no longer hunted people are less likely to come into contact with it.

**First aid: No local measures are known to relieve pain apart from an injection of local anaesthetic. Pressure—immobilisation is contraindicated as it will increase the pain. Hospital treatment, including systemic opiate therapy and antibiotics, may be required for severe cases.**

# 37 Scorpions

## Genus Urodacus

There are a number of species of scorpions throughout Australia and, like the centipedes, the further north, the larger and more potentially dangerous they become. Very small scorpions are quite often found in the undergrowth in suburban gardens.

Scorpions do not represent the danger to man in Australia that they do in Mexico, where some 1000 people die each year following scorpion stings. Indeed the only

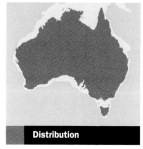

**Distribution**

probably death by a scorpion occurred many years ago in Western Australia. A baby girl was stung by a scorpion, which was then crushed beyond recognition by her father. The exact details are not known, other than that she died within 24 hours.

Scorpions sting with their tails. They are not aggressive but will attack if touched accidentally. The sting of the smaller scorpions is painful but soon wears off. The northern Australian scorpions may produce severe pain and swelling and the victim may not be able to work for several days.

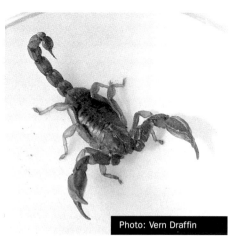

Photo: Vern Draffin

**First aid: Iced water may bring some relief. Severe cases may require hospitalisation and pain-killing drugs.**

# Jellyfish and Octopuses

# 38 Box Jellyfish *or* Sea Wasp

*Chironex fleckeri*

Since 1900 more than 70 people have died suddenly and painfully from Box Jellyfish stings in northern Australian waters. Many children have died within minutes of being stung. The average age of Box Jellyfish victims in Queensland is 14. No one should swim in tropical waters when the local people warn that the time of year and conditions of the sea are right for this deadly creature to come close to the shore.

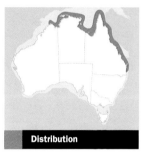

**Distribution**

The Box Jellyfish is found in coastal waters, creeks and rivers between the Tropics of Capricorn and Cancer. It is most likely to be encountered by swimmers during summer, but stings and even deaths have occurred at other times in the extreme north of Australia. On days that are hot and overcast but calm, the Box Jellyfish may move about in shallow water looking for small prawns. During the summer Wet when the rivers are muddy it is often very difficult to see the Box Jellyfish.

The Box Jellyfish has a box-shaped bell or body which may be as large as a two-gallon bucket (20 × 30 cm) and weigh more than 2 kg. Four bundles of up to 16 semi-transparent extendable tentacles stream out from four projections under the bell. The tentacles of adult specimens may stretch as far as 3 metres and can contract to one-quarter of their length. Thousands of millions of stinging capsules cover the tentacles and discharge venom via a penetrating thread into the skin of any creature which touches them. A second type of capsule produces a sticky substance which helps the tentacle stick to the victim. The Box Jellyfish jets along by ejecting water from its body cavity, and changes direction by altering the position of the cavity opening. It usually travels at less than 1 knot (about 2 km/h) but if alarmed can turn rapidly and perhaps reach a speed of 4 or 5 knots (about 7 to 9 km/h).

The Box Jellyfish uses its venom to catch its prey. It immobilises prawns which are then drawn into the body cavity for digestion. The venom contains 3 distinct ingredients. The major one causes death by shock to the heart and interference with the breathing mechanism. A minor ingredient attacks the victim's red blood cells. The venom also damages the skin where the capsules have penetrated. It has been estimated that an adult Box Jellyfish contains enough venom to kill at least 3 men. If the victim

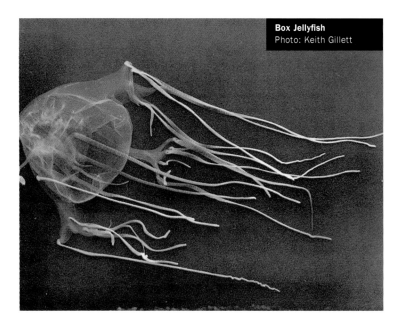

**Box Jellyfish**
Photo: Keith Gillett

survives but is not given antivenom, the part of the skin which has been stung ulcerates and often becomes permanently scarred and discoloured.

Often a child swims or wades across the trailing tentacles, tearing off long strips, many of which will instantly fire their stinging capsules. The threads and venom penetrate deep into the skin. The child screams, runs out of the water and collapses on the beach. Swollen lines, either purple or dark brown, appear over the body where it has been touched by the tentacles and it looks as if the victim has been whipped: the greater the area, the more severe the symptoms.

Antivenom to the Box Jellyfish venom is held by many life-saving and surf clubs in northern Australia. It is dangerous to swim at isolated beaches during summer months when this creature may be about. Swim only in patrolled areas when the local people say it is safe to do so.

 Box Jellyfish antivenom is used to treat stings.

 First Aid, see page 4

# 39 Chiropsalmus

## Chiropsalmus quadrigatus

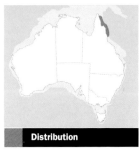

**Distribution**

**C**hiropsalmus is probably the next most potentially dangerous jellyfish after the Box Jellyfish. The first account in medical history of severe injuries caused by these large jellyfish was recorded in 1914. At least four types of jellyfish are known to cause human deaths. The other two are the Bluebottle (No. 38) and what are known as 'sand jellyfish' (genus *Stomolophus*). which is found around China.

Chiropsalmus is found only in the tropics, has a very wide distribution and inhabits both the Indian Ocean and the west Pacific Ocean. There are a number of difficult to distinguish species of *Chiropsalmus*. They are large jellyfish found in shallow coastal water as well as in the open sea and are quite powerful swimmers. They feed upon fish and shrimps.

A mature *Chiropsalmus quadrigatus* has a transparent bell or body with a diameter of 200 mm or more, and its tentacles may reach 1.5 metres in length. There are four bundles of seven tentacles in most specimens, and in live specimens these tentacles show narrow lavender bands of stinging cap-

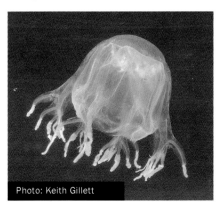

Photo: Keith Gillett

sules. The tentacles are very delicate, and usually break off and remain attached to clothing or the body if touched in the water.

Little is known of the actual properties of Chiropsalmus venom, but the symptoms are similar of those following stings by the Box Jellyfish. The same precautions should be taken to avoid contact with this jellyfish during summer months.

 Box Jellyfish antivenom neutralises the venom of the Chiropsalmus.

 First Aid, see page 4

# 40 Jimble

## Carybdea rastoni

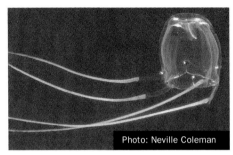
Photo: Neville Coleman

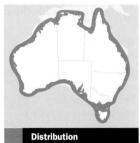
Distribution

The Jimble is one of a number of simple box-shaped, four-tentacled jellyfish which are widely distributed throughout the warmer waters of the world. The Jimble is found in coastal waters, bays and inlets around the whole of Australia, to a depth of 20 metres. It is very common in South Australia and south-western Australia. Jimbles like to swim in swarms, usually rising to the warmer surface of the sea in the early morning and evening. They are more common on cloudy days and are very difficult to see in the water. Sometimes swimmers notice the pink tentacles before they see the bell.

They are small creatures with a bell or body usually 2 cm across, but specimens 5 cm in diameter have been described. Jimbles have four tentacles which stretch out some 10 cm in length.

When the human skin makes contact with a Jimble tentacle, moderately severe local pain occurs which may last up to 2 hours. There is swelling and redness which may spread some 2.5 cm away from the actual sting site. The reaction lasts a long time and may still be visible a few weeks later. Sometimes blistering occurs in the area of the sting; sometimes there are ulcers and occasionally brown pigmentation may last for months. Occasionally a scar resembling the spokes of a wheel may radiate from the areas of maximum sting.

Although no deaths have so far been attributed to this creature, it is quite possible that a small child receiving multiple stings could become critically ill and even die.

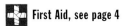 First Aid, see page 4

# 41 Irukandji

## *Carukia barnesi*

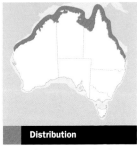
**Distribution**

For many years bathers near Cairns in Queensland complained of a peculiar type of sting. The illness produced by these stings was different from other marine stings. The immediate effects such as local pain and swelling were minor, but after about 30 minutes a headache, nausea, vomiting and pains in the joints developed and became progressively more severe. These symptoms were called type A sting or Irukandji stinging. (Irukandji was the name of an Aboriginal tribe living near Cairns.) The creature responsible for the stings was not captured until 1961 when two specimens were collected, identified, and given the name *Carukia barnesi* by Dr Southcott. The difficulty of finding specimens was overcome by the dedicated efforts of Dr Peter Fenner of Mackay, who has provided samples for The Australian Venom Research Unit since 1996.

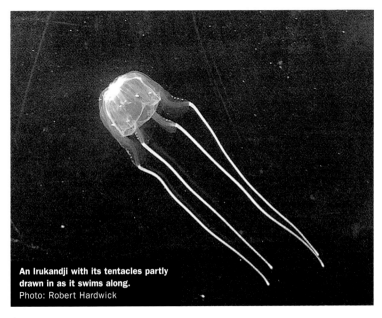
**An Irukandji with its tentacles partly drawn in as it swims along.**
Photo: Robert Hardwick

The Irukandji is found along the northern coastline of Australia, from Moreton Bay in Queensland to the Abrolhos Islands in Western Australia. It is much smaller than the more dangerous jellyfish. Its translucent bell or body is small (1.5 cm × 1 cm) and its four tentacles vary from 3 to 35 cm. The stinging capsules are seen as tiny red dots and these occur over the body as well as the tentacles.

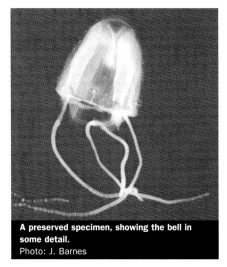

**A preserved specimen, showing the bell in some detail.**
Photo: J. Barnes

The victim usually does not see the Irukandji. The pain is felt within a few seconds of the sting and tends to decrease by 30 minutes. It is not usually severe but is enough to force the victim to leave the water. During the first 30 minutes some redness occurs around the area of contact and there may be slight swelling which rapidly goes down. The tentacles may be found to have stuck to the body. Between 5 minutes and as much as 2 hours after the sting, other symptoms may develop. Nausea, vomiting, sweating and agitation almost invariably occur. Abdominal pain is often caused by spasms of the muscles of the abdominal wall, and cramps may occur in the muscles of the limbs. Sometimes there are areas of numbness and tingling on the skin. There may be pains around the larger joints, especially shoulder and hip joints. As a general rule the temperature remains normal. Victims often have very high blood pressure which needs treatment in hospital with phentolamine, which also reduces the shaking and sweating.

No deaths are known to have been caused by these creatures, but the illness can be very difficult to manage at times and so the feasibility of an antivenom is under investigation. These jellyfish become a significant health problem when a number of bathers are affected at the same time. Like many marine dangers, this one may be avoided by not swimming when the authorities indicate that this potentially dangerous creature may be in the local waters.

 No antivenom has been developed at the time of writing.

 First Aid, see page 4

# 42 Blue-bottle _or_ Portuguese Man-of-war

_Physalia physalis_

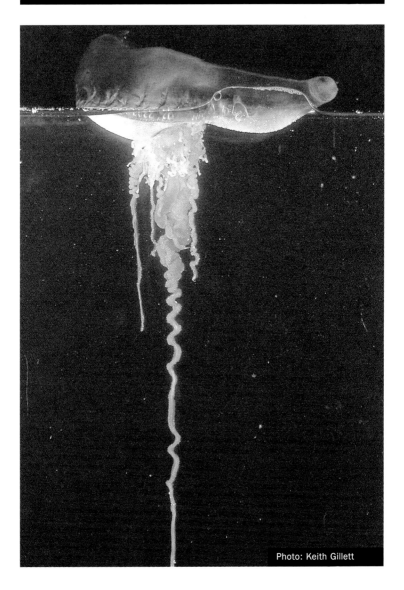

This species has a wide distribution in the warmer seas of the world. Occasionally it is found in large numbers either washed up on or in shallow water off popular beaches. Although it may give painful stings and cause beaches to be closed, it has caused no deaths in Australia, but has killed several people elsewhere. Being a surface swimmer, the Blue-bottle is a real danger to bathers, particularly when large numbers have gathered together. Tampering with stranded Blue-bottles on the beach may result in stings.

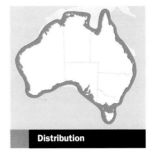

**Distribution**

The Blue-bottle has a gas-filled float to which a number of cysts and tentacles are attached. In fact each Blue-bottle consists of a number of individual animals which have developed special roles. One has become a float which keeps the group on the surface. Others are involved in reproduction, whilst the third group develops the polyps with their associated stinging tentacles and is responsible for the collection of food. Because of its float the Blue-bottle remains always on the surface of the sea. It uses its large float to catch the wind and it literally sails across the water. The tentacles consist of a bunch of short, frilled tentacles and a long trailing one used for fishing and also acting as a sea anchor. The long tentacle may grow to 10 metres and it is responsible for most of the stings.

Like the other important jellyfish poisons the Blue-bottle poison is believed to be a labile protein. In experimental animals it causes breathing failure and muscle weakness. Persons being stung by the creature experience sharp pain. Attempts to remove the tentacles may increase the number of stings. There may be single or multiple weals of different sizes and occasionally they occur in a zig-zag when the tentacle attaches to the skin only at certain points. Usually Blue-bottle weals have a ladder-like appearance due to the position of the stinging capsules on the tentacle. The severe pain lasts about 1 or 2 hours, and in bad cases it tends to spread sideways to surround joints if a limb has been stung and may move around the trunk if body stings have occurred. Severe pain may occur in the lymph nodes when the venom reaches them. Sometimes there are areas of bleeding at the site of the stings, and occasionally ulcers and permanent scarring may occur. The cornea of the eye can be damaged if it comes into contact with the tentacles of this creature. Some people develop a severe allergy to the poison of Blue-bottles and must take great care to avoid them.

**First Aid, see page 4**

# 43 Mauve Stinger *or* Mauve Blubber

*Pelagia noctiluca*

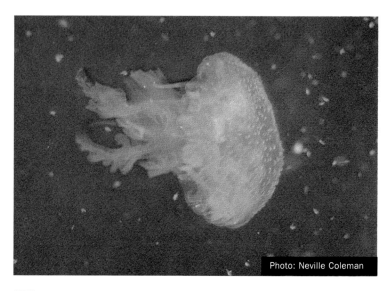

Photo: Neville Coleman

The Mauve Stinger or Mauve Blubber has a wide distribution in the oceans of the world. It is found both in tropical zones and in colder areas such as the north Atlantic and north Pacific Oceans.

This jellyfish is multicoloured. The bell or body of a mature specimen is usually some 12 cm in diameter and the upper surface has a number of warts. These warts and the tentacles contain stinging capsules.

The Mauve Stinger has not caused death in humans but has proved to be a nuisance when it appears in the sea, especially when sporting events such as major surfing championships are under way. Contact with its tentacles or bell can cause local pain, and on one occasion swimmers in a race near Brisbane who touched these jellyfish collapsed.

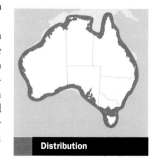

**Distribution**

# 44 Sea Blubber *or* Hairy Stinger

## Genus *Cyanea*

**H**airy jellyfish have a widespread distribution and are found in all Australian coastal waters. There are a number of species in this genus. Some have highly descriptive common names, like Hairy Stinger, Sea Nettle, Hairy Jelly and Lion's Mane.

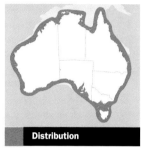

**Distribution**

They all have a flattened plate-like bell or body, the edge of which is turned inwards. A large number of delicate hairy tentacles trail downwards from 8 V-like clusters underneath the bell. The tentacles may easily become detached from the creature  and when separate can still inflict a painful sting. The bells may be more than 30 cm across in Australian waters, but in the cold Antarctic waters their size may be very much greater. It is believed that touching their dried tentacles on nets and fishing lines causes irritation.

Contact with the tentacles may produce a burning feeling which develops into a severe pain which may last up to an hour. Nausea and abdominal pains may develop. At times, profuse sweating, muscle cramps, and breathing difficulties occur. As with other jellyfish, injuries to the eye have occurred after contact with the tentacles. No deaths have been attributed to this creature.

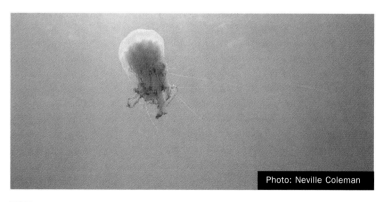

Photo: Neville Coleman

 First Aid, see page 4

93

# 45 Blue-ringed *or* Banded Octopus

## *Hapalochlaena maculosa, H. lunulata*

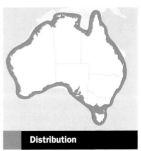

**Distribution**

There are two main species of *Hapalochlaena* octopuses, and both of them have been known to cause deaths in humans. The larger tropical species is *H. lunulata* and the common southern species is *H. maculosa*. Since the difference between the two species is only minor and more information is available about *H. maculosa*, this description is based on that species.

It is not clear where the boundary between the species occurs, but the Blue-ringed Octopus is present in all Australian coastal waters. It is extremely common, being found far more frequently in shallow water than any other type of octopus. It hunts at night and specimens are often washed up into small rock pools when the tide is rising, where they may bite any children or uninformed adults who pick them up.

The Blue-ringed Octopus is quite small and rarely exceeds 20 cm from the tip of one arm to the tip of another. In southern waters its maximum weight is about 90 g, the average mature specimen being 38 g. When undisturbed the octopus has dark brown to ochre bands over its arms and body with blue circles superimposed on these bands. When it is interfered with or taken out of the water the colours darken and the rings become a brilliant peacock blue. This dramatic and beautiful colour change, combined with the small size of the octopus, helps identification.

The diet of the Blue-ringed Octopus is mainly crabs. It catches these creatures after paralysing them with its poisonous saliva. The octopus has two large salivary or venom glands situated above its brain. A duct leads through the brain into its mouth parts, which terminate in a small parrot-like beak situated at the junction of its 8 arms. When hunting a crab, the octopus swims over it and sprays the poisonous saliva into the sea immediately surrounding it. The crab absorbs the poison and within a matter of minutes becomes paralysed. The octopus then descends upon it and devours it.

If the octopus is picked up by a human and, for example, carried on the forearm, it may at first attempt to escape, but if restrained it is likely to bite the skin with its small sharp beak. When this happens, its highly poisonous venom may be injected into the arm. Extensive studies of this venom

94

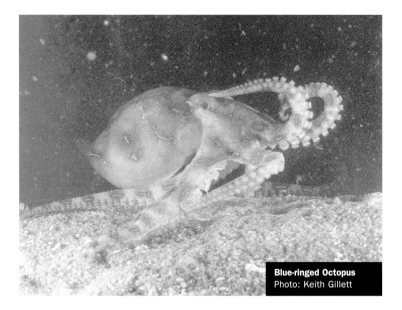

**Blue-ringed Octopus**
Photo: Keith Gillett

suggest that its main component is similar to the toxin (tetrodotoxin) that is present in the flesh of many poisonous fish, e.g. Toad or Puffer Fish. The poison interferes with the movement of impulses down the nerves of the body and results in a progressive paralysis. A mature Blue-ringed Octopus contains a large quantity of venom in its salivary glands. It has been estimated that sufficient venom may be present in one octopus to cause the paralysis of some 10 adult men.

When a human is bitten, the site of the bite may be relatively painless. If enough venom has been introduced, within a few minutes the victim will notice tingling sensations in the tongue and lips and will soon have difficulty seeing or speaking. Within 10 minutes they may have vomited and collapsed. Breathing may stop because of the paralysis.

If mouth-to-mouth resuscitation or some other type of artificial respiration is not given, the victim will become unconscious and eventually die from lack of oxygen.

*Remember*, this little creature is believed to be harmless in the water and will only bite humans if it is taken away from its natural environment. Like many other dangerous creatures it carries colours which allow it to be easily identified and which also flash a warning.

 **First aid:** If someone is bitten by one of these octopuses it is important to apply the direct pressure—immobilisation first aid (see pages 1–2) to the bitten area as soon as possible. If paralysis has occurred, adequate artificial ventilation may be required and this may have to be continued for some hours.

# Stinging Fish

# Introduction

Little is known about the venoms which are associated with the spines of the many kinds of stinging fish found in Australian waters. Furthermore, apart from the Stonefishes for which an antivenom is available, there is no specific treatment for any of these stings.

There are two problems posed by the venom of stinging fish. The severe pain which can develop after even what appears to be a trifling injury may produce a state of shock in the patient. It is very important in these cases to seek medical help to have the pain of the sting relieved. Of course, in many cases the severe pain is self-limiting and by 5 to 10 minutes is obviously declining. There are a number of drugs which may be used to reduce the pain. These range from the injection of local anaesthetics such as lignocaine to the injection of stronger pain killers such as pethidine; in some cases a regional nerve block may be considered. There is no doubt that stinging fish venom can cause great stress to its victims, and death may well occur if the person stung has already some physical weakness such as heart disease.

The other major problem which may follow marine stings is the development of infection. All stinging fish wounds, which may be quite deep and ragged, can be contaminated with foreign material. Patients have in fact died of tetanus some days after relatively minor marine stings.

Usually, stings by fish are easily avoided. Most fish should not be touched with the bare hands and it is particularly important to take care when landing fish either on a line or in nets at night. Many a pleasant fishing trip has been ruined by a fish using its defence mechanism effectively.

# 46 Bullrout *or* Kroki

## *Notesthes robusta*

The Bullrout has a number of other names, such as Scorpionfish, Wasp Fish and Rock Cod. It is commonly found in the estuaries and rivers of eastern Australia. It is slow moving and likes shallow, muddy waters. Stings occur when it is either trodden upon or accidentally kicked, or caught on fishing lines or in nets. This fish has been given the name Kroki because of the peculiar grunting sound it produces. If a number of the creatures are in one tank in a laboratory, their croaking can become a distraction.

The Bullrout has no scales and is usually a dull ochre colour; the maximum length reached is some 35 cm. It has 15 spines along the back, each associated with a pair of venom glands. Venomous spines are also found on the anal fin and the belly fins. Contact with the venomous spines results in intense and immediate pain. Over a few minutes the pain spreads away from the wound and may involve the whole of the envenomed limb. The lymph nodes draining the limb may become tender and swollen. In severe cases headache and vomiting can develop.

Some years ago one of the authors (SKS) received several Bullrout stings from a specimen in the laboratory. His finger only brushed the spine of the Bullrout and no mark on the skin could be seen with the naked eye, but severe pain developed instantly. The area of contact felt as though the head of a lighted match had flown off and was burning on the skin. The pain slowly faded over a 30-minute period and he was left wondering what it would be like to receive multiple deep stings from this innocuous looking creature.

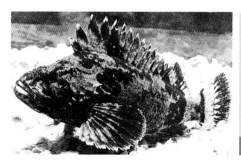

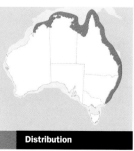

**Distribution**

 First Aid, see 'Stinging fish, especially stonefishes' page 5

# 47 Stonefish

There are a number of kinds of stonefish, which are the most dangerous of the venomous fishes. The important stonefish are *S. trachynis* (= *S. horrida*) and *S. verrucosa*. Two very descriptive names for stonefish are Nohu (the waiting one) and Warty-ghoul.

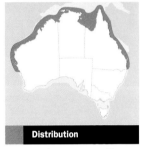

**Distribution**

Stonefish are found around two-thirds of the coastline of Australia, extending from Moreton Bay in Queensland to 500 km north of Perth. Although Stonefish are quite common, they are usually not seen unless they are either very carefully looked for or come into contact with the human foot or hand. They inhabit coral reefs and shallow mud flats and usually lie covered with slime and with algae attached, well camouflaged on the bottom of the sea from where they may suck small passing fish into their very large mouths. Often they are partially buried in the sand. Their mouths snap open and shut very quickly.

The stonefish is a heavily built, cumbersome creature which may grow to a length of 47 cm. It has 13 sharp spines along the back, each associat-

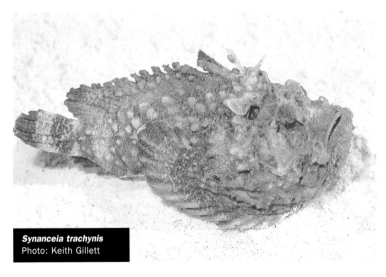

**Synanceia trachynis**
Photo: Keith Gillett

ed with 2 venom glands. The spines and their associated venom play no part in its feeding habits. If a human stands on a stonefish it is relatively easy for the sharp spines to penetrate deep into the foot of the victim (even through sandshoes or thongs). As the spine enters the flesh a combination of venom and actual portions of the venom glands may be deposited in the tissues. The victim immediately feels excruciating pain, the severity of which is in proportion to the size and number of spines which have injured the foot or hand. Stonefish venom contains a number of ingredients, some of which cause severe local pain and tissue damage. One of these can cause damage to the muscles of the heart some hours after the actual injury.

For many years, all reported cases of stonefish stings have been on the hands or the feet of the victim. Either the fish has been grasped in the hand when it was brought up on a fishing line or it has been trodden on by a person with unprotected feet.

Stonefish antivenom became available in 1959 and has been found to reduce dramatically all effects of the venom, including the pain. All cases of significant injury should receive antivenom.

Australians regularly suffer Stonefish stings when holidaying on Pacific islands. Special care should be taken at these resorts as usually no Stonefish antivenom is available and permanent damage to the hands or feet may occur.

 Stonefish antivenom is available to treat stings.

 First Aid, see 'Stinging fish, especially stonefishes' page 5

# 48 Butterfly Cod

*Pterois volitans*

The genus *Pterois* includes a number of species of beautifully coloured fish, which have common names such as Zebra Fish, Firecod, Lion Fish and Red-fire Fish. They may grow as long as 42.5 cm and weigh 1 kg.

Butterfly Cod may be found as far south as Perth and Sydney and are common in shallow water around rocks and coral reefs. They are curious

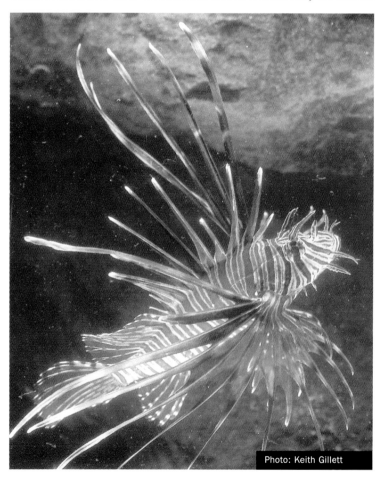

Photo: Keith Gillett

creatures and frequently approach divers, usually in pairs, with their 13 stinging spines projected forward as a defence. Each spine is associated with a pair of delicate venom glands and the venom passes to the tip of the spine through a narrow duct.

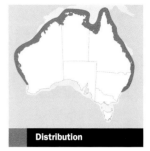

**Distribution**

If a person is stung by the spines of this fish, severe pain occurs instantly. The pain increases in severity over a few minutes, often becoming so extreme that the victim weeps and becomes greatly distressed. It may last several days but usually subsides after a few hours. The puncture wound itself is generally numb and is surrounded by a bluish discolouration and swelling. The more stings inflicted, the more severe the general symptoms. Usually the lymph nodes draining the stung area become swollen and tender. Vomiting, fever and sweating sometimes occur, but the most significant effect of the venom is the distress and severe pain which appears out of proportion to the injury which has been inflicted. No deaths are known to have occurred in Australia following stings by this creature, but they have been reported overseas.

In recent years, Butterfly Cod have become increasingly popular as aquarium fish and, as a result, injuries from their stinging spines have become more common. Often the buying public are not even warned that contact with the spines may cause a painful injury.

First Aid, see 'Stinging fish, especially stonefishes' page 5

# *49* Catfish

## Genera *Plotosus, Cnidoglanis and Arius*

**C**atfish can be quite a severe threat to fishermen, particularly those fishing at night who may not be able clearly to identify the fish they have caught. There are a number of kinds of catfish distributed around Australia and they can all inflict a moderate injury. The common names of some are confusing: for example, in New South Wales, South Australia and Western Australia, the Estuary Catfish (*Cnidoglanis macrocephalus*) is called the Cobbler, which is also the name given to a different species of stinging fish found in South Australia and Victoria (*Gymnapistes marmoratus*) (No. 60). Other names for catfish are the Eel-tailed Catfish (*Plotosus lineatus*) and

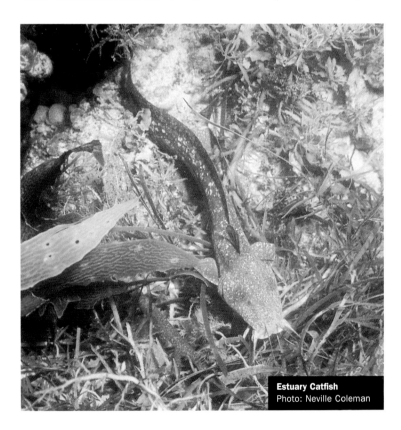

**Estuary Catfish**
Photo: Neville Coleman

Cattie. These fish are called catfish because of the long whiskers around their lips.

Catfish are frequently found is estuaries, seagrass meadows, rivers, mud flats, reef and coral reefs at a depth of 1 to 40 metres, and are often caught in fishing nets. They live on worms, small shellfish and sea snails. They vary in length, ranging from 5 cm in some species to 1 metre.

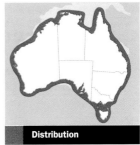

**Distribution**

Catfish have a long venomous spine on the back and two spines on the side or chest. Their spines are extremely sharp and easily penetrate the skin. It is particularly dangerous to try and hold a catfish as the three spines will spring out vertically and penetrate one's hand. There are delicate venom glands which run the length of the spine. The venom causes immediate, severe pain like the venoms of other stinging fish, and the severity of the pain is often far greater than one would expect from such an injury. It usually does not last more than several hours, but sometimes it may persist for 24 hours.

No deaths have been reported in Australia following catfish stings.

First Aid, see 'Stinging fish, especially stonefishes' page 5

# 50 Surgeonfish

## *Acanthurus dussumieri*

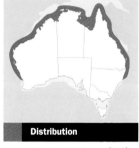

**Distribution**

The Surgeonfish is also known as the Doctorfish, the Tang and the Spinetail. Apart from injuring fishermen who have just caught it, it has occasionally attacked people when they and the fish were in the same confined area. It is edible but may occasionally be poisonous if it has devoured smaller fish which were carrying the poison ciguatoxin.

The Surgeonfish is capable of causing deep lacerations by the rapid movement of sharp spines near its tail. The speed with which these injuries can be inflicted have led to the common names given to the fish. Its spine may be venomous as the pain produced by the incisions is greater than might be expected. In fact, it may last hours or even days.

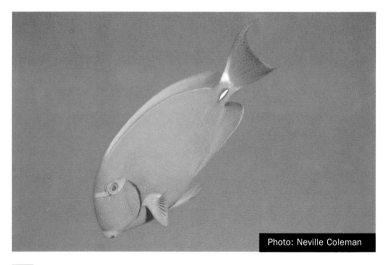

Photo: Neville Coleman

**First aid:** Bleeding may be a problem and it is important to apply firm pressure to the lacerated area as soon as possible. The victim must also be quickly removed from the water.

# 51 Old Wife

## *Enoplosus armatus*

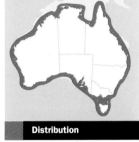

**Distribution**

The Old Wife is also known as the Zebra Fish. It is widely distributed around the Australian coast and is frequently seen but rarely hooked as it swims around jetties and wharves. It lives on seagrass meadows or reefs at a depth of 5 to 50 metres. Generally, it is not solitary and can be found in pairs or groups which separate when disturbed.

Mature specimens may be as long as 25 cm. Its zebra-like markings may be brown or black and the backs of the hind and anal rays are bright red and the tail pink. It eats small shellfish and worms. The name 'Old Wife' is supposedly due to the creature's habit of grinding its teeth and 'grumbling'.

It has a number of finely pointed venomous spines on the back which inflict a sharp pain if they penetrate the skin. Generally the injuries are mild, but occasionally severe pain may extend over the whole of the stung limb and the victim may develop vomiting and a headache. Painful stings can be avoided by not handling this creature when it has been caught in fishing nets or speared by divers.

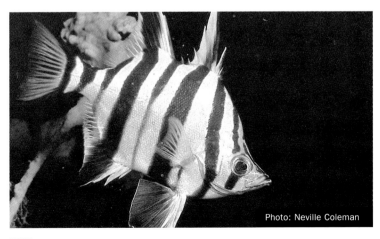

Photo: Neville Coleman

 First Aid, see 'Stinging fish, especially stonefishes' page 5

# 52 Frogfish

*Halophryne diemensi*

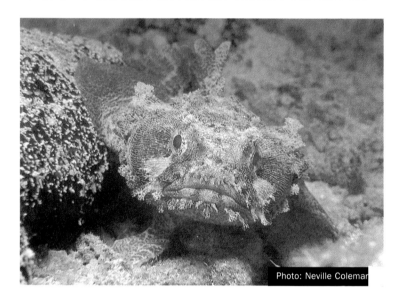

Photo: Neville Coleman

This strange looking fish is also known as the Banded Frogfish or the Bastard Stonefish. It is common among coral and rocks in tropical waters where it grows to a maximum length of 25 cm. It has frilly side fins but no scales. Its colouring ranges from violet to purplish-black, pearly grey or lilac below with crossbands or mottlings of a lighter colour speckled with spots or dots. Sometimes it is scarlet or orange-brown

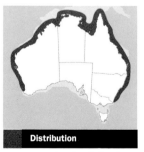

**Distribution**

above. It is a floppy-looking fish which can survive on dry land for long periods and may be found creeping over mud and slime. It has two spines on the back and two on the sides, which are considered to be venomous. Its sting causes severe local pain and occasional mild general symptoms; no other details are known of the injuries produced by this creature.

 First Aid, see 'Stinging fish, especially stonefishes' page 5

# 53 Bearded Ghoul Chinese Ghoul

*Inimicus caledonicus*
*Inimicus sinensis*

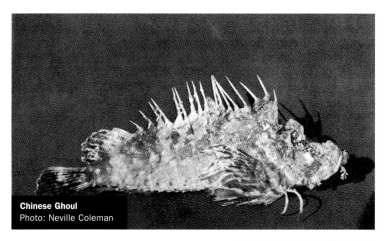

**Chinese Ghoul**
Photo: Neville Coleman

This particular genus contains several extremely spiky and strange-looking species. Another name for the Bearded Ghoul is the Demon Stinger. It is quite common in the waters of Queensland where, on occasions, it has been reported to have attacked underwater photographers. Very often it is caught by prawn trawlers.

It grows to about 33 cm in length, and is black or brown above, passing into darker

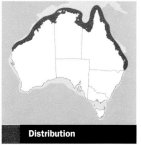

**Distribution**

brown or light brown on the sides and usually freckled with blackish brown. It has a yellowish-brown belly. The Bearded Ghoul has about 17 very long spines on the back which can cause painful injuries. A sting from a Bearded Ghoul may be painful for hours; the victim may become quite ill and take several days to recover fully. A special feature of its stings may be the occurrence of swelling in the limb that has been stung. A state of shock may develop. Relief of pain is very important. Sometimes patients sleep for several days after suffering a severe sting by this creature.

 First Aid, see 'Stinging fish, especially stonefishes' page 5

# 54 Goblinfish

## *Glyptauchen panduratus*

**T**his fish is also known as the Saddlehead. It is found further south than most of the stinging fish previously described. Other species in the genus inhabit the south and south-east coasts.

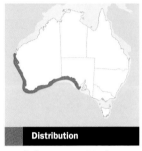

**Distribution**

The Goblinfish grows to a length of some 25 cm. It has 17 spines on the back which are closely webbed. Contact with these spines can produce severe pain and the patient may become shocked and collapse. The pain appears out of proportion to the size of the injury. Nothing is known about the properties of Goblinfish venom.

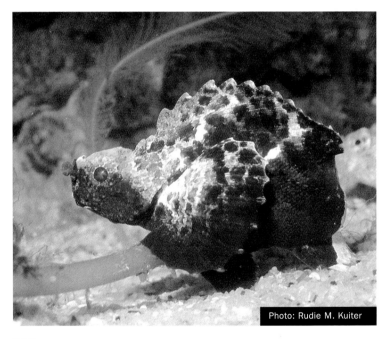

Photo: Rudie M. Kuiter

 First Aid, see 'Stinging fish, especially stonefishes' page 5

# 55 Red Rock Cod Chained Scorpionfish

*Scorpaena cardinalis*
*Scorpaena papillosus*

These fish are also known as the Cardinal Scorpionfish and Red Scorpion Cod, and by the delightful name Mouth Almighty. They grow to some 38 cm in length and are quite common in the waters around the south-eastern parts of Australia as far north as Queensland. They like rocky reefs from 4 to 40 metres deep and feed on small fish and shellfish. They are frequently caught by fishermen who in turn may be stung by the 13

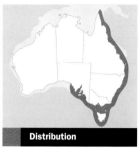

**Distribution**

sharp spines on the back or the spines around the head. Scratches from these spines may be tender for days. Usually the hand is injured and the pain may spread up the arm and cover the chest within an hour. There may also be general symptoms such as pallor, vomiting or collapse.

The flesh of this fish is good to eat, but the greatest care should be taken when it is being filleted. Some sensible fishermen refuse to have it pulled into their boats.

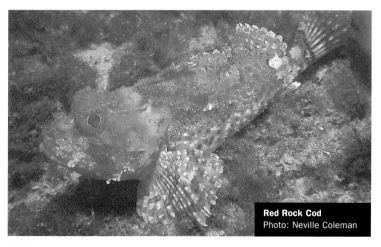

**Red Rock Cod**
Photo: Neville Coleman

 First Aid, see 'Stinging fish, especially stonefishes' page 5

## Siganus spinus, S. lineatu.

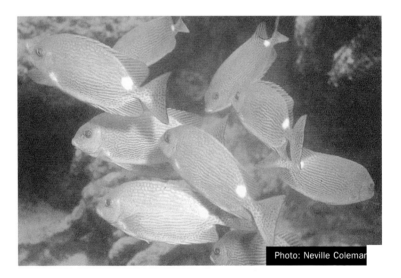

Photo: Neville Coleman

These fish look somewhat like the Surgeonfish (No. 50). *S. spinus* is also known as Black Trevally, Black Spinefoot, the Stinging Bream, the Mi-Mi, and also by the perverse name Happy Moments. It is usually found in schools feeding upon seaweed on reefs in northern Queensland.

The average length of a mature specimen is 20 cm. It is a slate-blue colour with long yellow lines and spots on the sides. The face

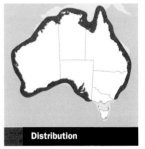

**Distribution**

and cheeks are yellow with bright blue lines, and there are yellow spots below the last rays on the back. Rabbit fish have 13 venomous spines on the back and a number of pelvic and anal spines. The first spine on the back is the one which usually inflicts the injury as the fish tends to lower its head and engage with this spine when provoked. Like many other stinging fish, the pain produced is greater than the size of the injury would suggest.

 First Aid, see 'Stinging fish, especially stonefishes' page 5

# 57 Rat Fish

## *Hydrolagus lemures*

This strange-looking fish, which can grow to over half a metre in length, is sometimes caught by trawlers fishing in deep temperate waters.

It has a large spine on the back with paired venom glands which extend to the tip of the spine. As well as this quite vicious spine, the fish has a well-developed dental plate capable of causing extensive bites. Although stings by this fish are rare they

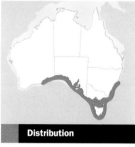

**Distribution**

may be quite dangerous because, apart from the introduction of venom, the tissue damage caused by such a large spine can be serious. Deep and ragged wounds are quite likely to become infected.

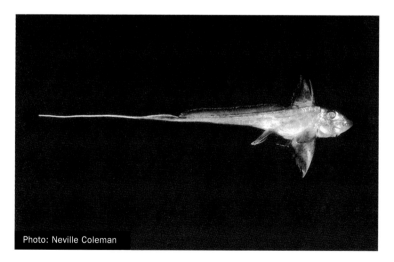

Photo: Neville Coleman

 First Aid, see 'Stinging fish, especially stonefishes' page 5

# 58 Flatheads

## Family Platycephalidae

**F**latheads are probably one of the commonest causes of pain and distress among amateur fishermen.

About 30 species of flatheads are found in Australian waters in a variety of habitats, varying between estuaries and bays to the continental shelf. They are difficult to see as their colour is similar to that of their surroundings. They are bottom-dwelling fish and like burying themselves in sand with

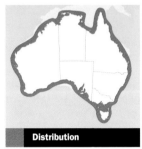

**Distribution**

just their eyes exposed; even these are often covered with sandy-coloured flaps. Their body is very compressed—to extremes in some species. The head is often armed with large spines and ridges; the mouth is large and a few species possess fair sized teeth. They are fish of moderate size; the Dusky Flathead (*Platycephalus fuscus*) may grow to over a metre in length, but most southern species average about 50 cm maximum.

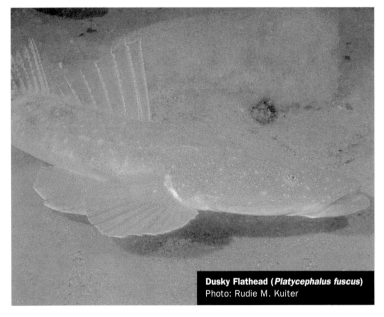

**Dusky Flathead (*Platycephalus fuscus*)**
Photo: Rudie M. Kuiter

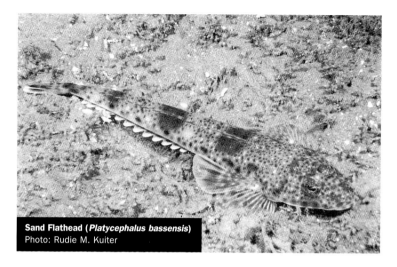

**Sand Flathead (*Platycephalus bassensis*)**
Photo: Rudie M. Kuiter

All species of flathead are excellent eating. In southern waters they are very important to the fishing industry, and both professional and regular amateur fishermen know about the risk of being wounded by the spines on the head and particularly the double spines on the lower side. However, the occasional fisherman may not know about them.

First Aid, see page 5. It is reported that rubbing slime from the skin of the fish into the wound may relieve the pain but there is no proof of this. Probably the pain subsides at its own rate regardless of treatment. Minor bleeding should be encouraged to clean the wound and although the pain may persist for some time no serious effects are known.

# 59 Fortescue

*Centropogon australis*

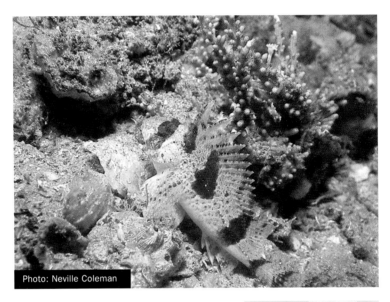

Photo: Neville Coleman

This fish, which is also known as the Wasp Fish, does not grow larger than 15 cm. It is common in the estuaries of eastern Australia. The Marbled Fortescue (*C. marmoratus*) is similar but smaller and is especially common in the waters of Moreton Bay in Queensland. Both the spines of the back and those of the fins are venomous.

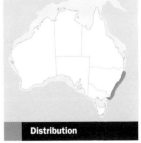

Distribution

Both species are often caught in nets and on lines, and even very small specimens can cause painful stings. The signs and symptoms of Fortescue stings are similar to those of other stinging fish. It is a special danger to uninformed skin divers, who may be tempted to catch it as it is a very slow-moving fish. Fishermen are sometimes stung when they accidentally touch a Fortescue while collecting shellfish for bait.

 First Aid, see 'Stinging fish, especially stonefishes' page 5

# 60 South Australian Cobbler

*Gymnapistes marmoratus*

There are a number of kinds of cobblers found all around Australia, but perhaps the most important is the South Australian Cobbler, also known as the Scorpionfish or Soldierfish. In Western Australia the name 'cobbler' is sometimes given to catfish (No. 49).

The South Australian Cobbler usually lives on the bottom of the sea on rocky reefs, in mud, seagrass meadows, sand and rubbish,

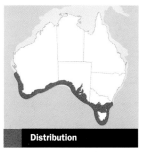

**Distribution**

and moves about at night. In summer it inhabits shallow waters less than 20 metres deep, moving to the depths in winter. The maximum length is 23 cm. It looks rather like the Fortescue (No. 59), but may easily be told apart since it lacks scales on both the body and the head.

The South Australian Cobbler has 13 venomous spines on the back and 3 anal spines, a breast spine and 4 spines around the mouth. They are all capable of producing a venomous sting which causes exquisite pain. Fishermen pulling in their nets in southern waters at night are in particular danger. It seems possible that the death of one man with a heart condition was brought on by the severe pain and shock he experienced when he accidentally grasped a Cobbler in his hand.

Preliminary work on the venom of the South Australian Cobbler indicates it has a wide number of different actions in tissues apart from the ability to cause pain.

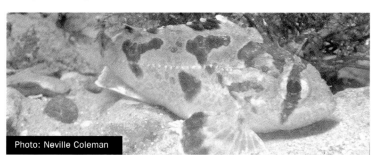

Photo: Neville Coleman

 First Aid, see 'Stinging fish, especially stonefishes' page 5

# Other Sea Creatures

# 61  Stingrays

**A** large number of stingrays are found in Australian waters. They are the largest of the venomous fish, although in practice the damage done by the penetration of the stinging barb is greater than that caused by the actual venom.

Stingrays tend to feed on the seabed and lie there motionless. When someone treads on them or swims low over them they respond by a sudden vertical thrust of the

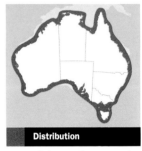

**Distribution**

tail which drives the spine into the victim. There is a delicate skin over the Stingray's serrated spine which is broken at the time of penetration, and venom may enter the wound by passing along grooves running along the spine. Because of the size of the spine and the strength of the creature the injury can be extremely serious. For example, two Australians are known to have died following heart injuries inflicted by Stingrays.

The commonest site for a sting is the leg. Apart from the immediate danger of physical damage to the body the most usual complication is infection. In particular, tetanus may develop after a stingray injury and this may lead to death some days after the actual sting. Sometimes a chronic infection may develop due to portions of the sting remaining in the wound.

### Duckbill Ray                    *Aetobatus narinari*

The Duckbill Ray, also called the Spotted Eagle Ray or Beaked Eagle Ray, is found in the warmer waters of Australia. It is a very beautiful creature, being covered with many white or grey or even blue spots. The tail is very long and thin and the actual spine is short and is situated near the base of the tail.

### Black Stingray                  *Dasyatis thetidis*

Also called the Black Stingray, Smooth Stingray or Thorntail Stingray, this true stingray grows to be the largest in the world, with a width of up to 2 metres and a length of 4.2 metres.

## Butterfly Ray
*Gymnura australis*

Butterfly or Rat-tailed Rays are found in tropical waters. Their sting is quite stumpy, as is their actual tail. Sometimes they have no sting.

## Common Stingaree
*Urolophus testaceus*

This species is also called the Common Stingray, Sandyback Stingray, Greenback Stingray or Round Stingray. It is found all around the coast of Australia, both in shallow waters and in the deep sea. The young are born live, i.e. eggs are not laid. The adult is relatively small for a stingray, growing to only 80 cm in length.

## Bat Ray
*Myliobatis australis*

Bat Rays, also called Eagle Rays, are often seen in aquariums where their graceful swimming movements are greatly admired. They are found in all seas around Australia and may grow to a width of more than 1.3 metres. The lateral flaps of these stingrays are often sold as 'skate' at fish markets.

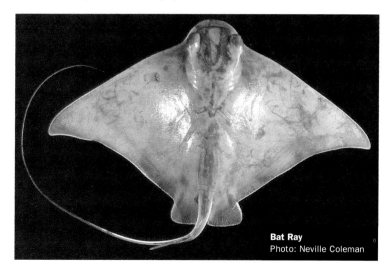

**Bat Ray**
Photo: Neville Coleman

 First Aid, see 'Stinging fish, especially stonefishes' page 5

# 62 Cone shells

## Genus *Conus*

Since 1705 it has been known that cone shells are capable of causing serious injury to humans. There are a wide variety of cone shells but only some of those found in tropical waters are considered dangerous. There has been one proven case of death following a sting by a cone shell in Australia and this was made by a Geographer Cone. The following cone shells (listed in decreasing order of their probable degree of danger)

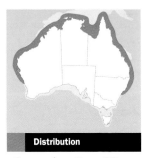

**Distribution**

are known to be highly dangerous to humans: Geographer Cone (*C. geographus*), Cloth of Gold Cone (*C. textile*) (also called Textile or Woven Cone), Tulip Cone (*C. tulipa*), Marbled Cone (*C. marmoreus*), Court Cone (*C. aulicus*) and Pearled Cone (*C. omaria*). Studies of the Striated Cone (*C. striatus*) suggest that it carries insufficient venom.

Cone shells are so called because they are conical or cylindrical in shape. During the day they bury themselves in the sand and at night emerge and crawl around in search of food. Cones are carnivorous; some species feed on small fish, others on snails and some upon worms. The victim of a cone shell is speared and then paralysed with small teeth or harpoons which have been soaked in poison. These little harpoons have a number of barbs and are hollow. When the prey is sighted, the harpoon is pushed out like a dart through a long snout into the target. Venom may be pumped into the prey through the harpoon, which usually remains gripped by the cone shell though it can be detached. In this way, passing fish may be speared, captured and then eaten. The harpoons are usually 1 cm in length and are made of hard, bone-like material. Each creature possesses a number of them. Studies suggest various cone shell venoms have widely different actions. However, the overall effect is to cause paralysis of the major muscles of the body.

People who pick up these beautiful shells may be in great danger if the shells are still occupied by the original inhabitants. Even holding one by the broad blunt end may not guarantee safety because the snout with its associated dart can extend from the narrow end to near the base. A person impaled by one these darts may feel immediate pain which soon gives way to numbness. If a large dose of venom has been injected the next sensation is tingling around the lips and mouth. Soon breathing may become

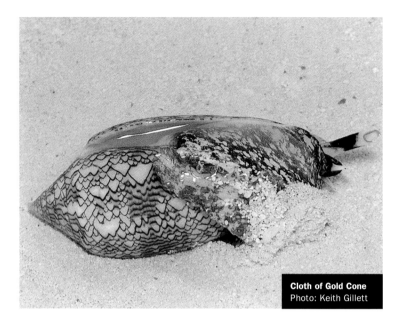

**Cloth of Gold Cone**
Photo: Keith Gillett

difficult and the victim may lapse into coma. Unless this severe paralysis is treated with prolonged mouth-to-mouth resuscitation the patient may soon die. There is no antivenom available for any of the cone shell venoms.

On Hayman Island in 1935 a young man picked up a live cone shell which was later identified as a Geographer Cone. He was stung in the palm of the hand and just a small puncture mark was visible. There was no pain at any time. A feeling of slight numbness started at once, and some 10 minutes later he complained of stiffness about the lips. After 20 minutes his sight was blurred, and in 30 minutes his legs were paralysed. In 60 minutes he was unconscious and appeared to be in a deep coma. He died 5 hours after receiving the sting.

 **First aid:** Immediately apply the pressure–immobilisation method (see pages 1–2). Prolonged mouth-to-mouth resuscitation may be required. It is possible now with modern intensive-care methods for a victim to survive the paralysis if they reach help early enough.

# 63 Port Jackson Shark

*Heterodontus portusjackson*

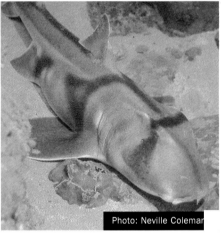

Photo: Neville Coleman

Although originally thought to be found only in Port Jackson in New South Wales, this extremely primitive shark has a very wide distribution around the temperate parts of Australia and New Zealand. Its other names are Oyster Crusher, Bullhead, Dogshark and Doggie. It lives on the bottom of the sea on rocky reefs, in sand, mud or seagrass meadows at a depth of 8 to 200 metres. In winter it comes into shallow waters to breed. It crunches up oysters with its powerful jaws, and also eats fish and sea urchins.

It grows to 1.4 metres long and is one of the few venomous sharks known, having a poisonous spine at the front of each of the 2 fins on its back. When hooked on a fishing line or caught by a spear fisherman, the twisting motions of its body may bring the spine into contact with the skin of the fisherman or skin diver and a few centimetres of the spine can enter the flesh. Apart from making a ragged and potentially infected wound, the spine produces marked local pain and local muscle weakness which may last several hours. The muscle weakness may involve the whole of the limb.

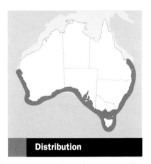

**Distribution**

 First Aid, see 'Stinging fish, especially stonefishes' page 5

# 64 Glaucus

## *Glaucus atlanticus*

The Glaucus is also known as the Sea Lizard. The creature is often found floating with its underside towards the sky. This is usually an attractive blue, while the back is a shiny white. The creature is seldom longer than 3 cm. The Glaucus 'recycles' other creatures' stinging capsules. They may be tiny stinging capsules from minute marine creatures or larger stinging capsules such as those from the Blue-bottle.

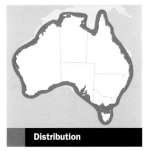

**Distribution**

Contact with the Glaucus may result in injury if the stinging capsules are triggered off. Its severity will depend on the number of stinging capsules fired and, of course, their origin. The wound will not show the orderly lines of a normal injury from stinging capsules but the marks will be scattered over the area of actual contact. Usually a blotchy red patch appears over the sting and both the swelling and the pain increase for some 15 minutes and then subside.

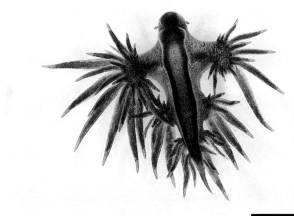

Photo: Keith Gillett

 First Aid, see 'Other Jellyfish Stings', page 4

# Further Reading

Cogger, H.G. (1996) *Reptiles and Amphibians of Australia*. Frenchs Forest, NSW: Reed Books.

Covacevich, J., Davie, P. and Pearn, J. (eds) (1987) *Toxic Plants and Animals: A Guide for Australia*. Brisbane: Queensland Museum.

Edmonds, C. (1989) *Dangerous Marine Creatures*. Frenchs Forest, NSW: Reed Books.

Gow, G.F. (1993) *Graeme Gow's Complete Guide to Australian Snakes*. Sydney: Cornstalk Publishing.

Hawdon, G. and Winkel, K.D. (1997) Venomous marine creatures. *Australian Family Physician* **26**: 1369–74.

Hawdon, G. and Winkel, K.D. (1997) Spider bite: a rational approach. *Australian Family Physician* **26**: 1380–85.

Hawdon, G. and Winkel, K.D. (1997) Could this be snake bite? *Australian Family Physician* **26**: 1386–91.

Mascord, R. (1983) *Australian Spiders in Colour*. Sydney: A.H. & A.W. Reed.

Mirtschin, P. and Davis, R. (1992) *Snakes of Australia: Dangerous and Harmless*. Melbourne: Hill of Content.

Shine, R. (1993) *Australian Snakes: A Natural History*. Australia: Reed Books.

Sutherland, S.K. (1983) *Australian Animal Toxins. The Creatures, their Toxins and Care of the Poisoned Patient*. Melbourne: Oxford University Press.

Sutherland, S.K. and King, K. (1991) *Management of snakebite in Australia*. Royal Flying Doctor Service of Australia Monograph Series No. 1.

Underhill, D. (1987) *Australia's Dangerous Creatures*. Sydney: Readers' Digest.

Weigel, J. (1990) *Guide to the Snakes of South-East Australia*. Gosford, NSW: Australian Reptile Park.

Williamson, J.A., Fenner, P.J., Burnett, J.W. and Rifkin, J.F. (eds) (1996) *Venomous and Poisonous Marine Animals: A Medical and Biological Handbook*. Sydney: University of New South Wales Press.

# Index

If doctors require appropriate consultants, they can be contacted via the Poisons Information Centres (**131126** Australia wide). Doctors may also contact the medical staff of the Australian Venom Research Unit directly on **(03) 9483-8204** or CSL Ltd on **(03) 9389-1911**.

*Note: entries in italics indicate incidental mentions of the subject in the text.*

allergy and anaphylaxis, 8–9
American Brown Recluse, 74
American Diamond Rattlesnake,
    venom of, 16
antivenoms, 7–8
ants, 54–5
*Arius* (genus), 104–5
Australian Paralysis Tick, 74–5

Banded Frogfish, 108
Banded Octopus, 94–5
Banded Sea Snake, 52
Bastard Stonefish, 108
Bat Ray, 120
Beaked Sea Snake, 52
bees, 56–7 (*see also* allergy and
    anaphylaxis)
Black House Spider, 73
Black Snake,
    Blue-bellied, 34
    Red-bellied, 30
black snakes, 30–5
Black Spinefoot, 112
Black Stingray, 120
Black Trevally, 112
Black Window Spider, 73
Blubber,
    Mauve, 92
    Sea, 93

Blue Ant (wasp), 59
Blue Mountains Funnel-web
    Spider, 68
Blue-bellied Black Snake, 34
Blue-bottle, 90–1, *125*
Blue-ringed Octopus, 94–5
Box Jellyfish, 84–5
Bream, Stinging, 112
Broad-headed Snake, 46–7
Brown Recluse, *see* Fiddleback
    Spider
Brown Snake,
    Common (Eastern), 22–3
    False King, 33
    King, 32–3, *35*
    Speckled, 27
    Western, 24–5
brown snakes, 22–7
Brown Widow Spider, 64
Bull Ant, 54–5
Bullhead, 120
Bullrout, 99
Butterfly Cod, 102–3
Butterfly Ray, 120

Cardinal Scorpionfish, 111
Catfish, 104–5
Cattle Tick, 74
centipedes, 78–9
Chained Sorpionfish, 111
Chiropsalmus, 86–7
Clarence River Snake, 42–3